COCONUT OIL

FOR BEGINNERS

YOUR COCONUT OIL MIRACLE GUIDE

HEALTH CURES, BEAUTY, WEIGHT LOSS, AND DELICIOUS RECIPES

Rockridge Press

CONTENTS

INTRODUCTION TO COCONUT OIL

Welcome to the world of coconut oil! If you're looking for information about the latest, greatest ingredient to hit the health-food and natural-healing scenes, then you've come to the right place. But be prepared, because coconut oil is nothing new; it's been around for centuries but was demonized in Western society along with every other form of saturated fat back in the 1960s. Fortunately for us, those who knew that all saturated fats weren't actually bad for you didn't stop using coconut oil.

The coconut has been a staple crop for thousands of years throughout coastal regions of North and South America, Asia, Africa, as well as in the Pacific Islands. The oil, in particular, has so many uses that an exhaustive list would take up the next four pages. The ones that we're going to be focusing on throughout the following chapters are:

- Health
- Beauty
- Weight loss
- Cooking

This book presents a brief history of coconut oil, along with what its traditional uses have been. It also explains exactly why coconut oil shouldn't be lumped in with other "bad" saturated fats, and it covers the different extraction and packaging methods so you know what to look for when you go out to buy your own. Finally, this book shares some marvelous recipes for meals, soaps, conditioners, massage oils, and even deodorants that are made from this incredible oil.

Are you ready to get to it? If so, then let's talk coconut!

SECTION ONE

Coconut Oil Basics

- **Chapter 1:** A Brief History of Coconut Oil

- **Chapter 2:** A Shopper's Guide to Coconut Oil

- **Chapter 3:** The Science of Coconut Oil

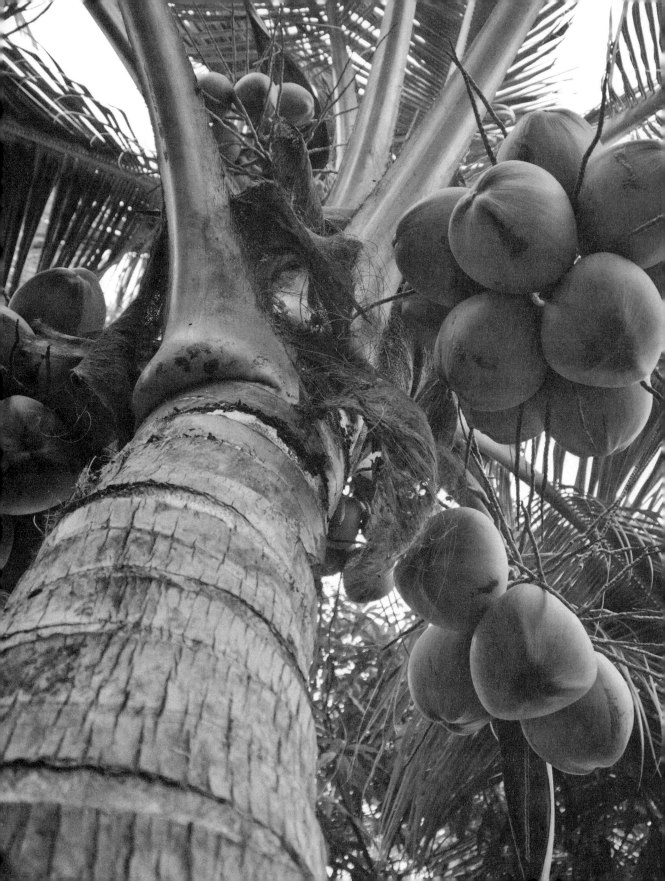

A BRIEF HISTORY OF COCONUT OIL

Known also as the Tree of Life, the coconut palm's origin is unknown. Many botanists, however, lean toward it being an Old World plant originally from Polynesia or the Indian Archipelago because there are more varieties of palms in those places than anywhere else. Nonetheless, the true "roots" of the tree are a mystery. What we do know is that the earliest written reference to a coconut comes from a fifth-century traveling merchant and monk named Cosmas Indicopleustes.

Cosmas described the trees and referred to the "India nuts" in text and in pictures when describing Sri Lanka and other places. Since he described the harvesting and use of the coconuts, it's safe to assume that they predate the fifth century by quite a bit; otherwise the procedures wouldn't have already been established.

Who Grows Coconuts?

Though coconut palms are present in just about every tropical coastal area that you can imagine, concentrated production and harvesting occur in significant proportions in only a handful of countries. However, in places where coconut harvest does occur, it often accounts for a pretty big chunk of the local economy. The countries that produce and export the most coconut oil are:

- Philippines
- Indonesia
- India

- Vietnam
- Mexico
- Papua New Guinea
- Thailand
- Sri Lanka
- Malaysia
- Mozambique
- Côte d'Ivoire
- Tanzania
- Nigeria
- Samoa
- Ghana

The first five countries account for the vast majority of coconut oil production, but quality products come from the other exporters as well. Also, these are just the countries that export it; many others produce it in small quantities for personal or community use.

Cool Coconut Fact

Coconut palms grow in tropical regions as far north as Hawaii and as far south as Madagascar, and it takes from nine to twelve months for a coconut to mature.

Historical Uses of Coconut Oil

Because they're used for so many purposes beyond simple nutrition, coconuts are known as functional foods. For centuries, people from coastal Asia, the Pacific Islands, Mexico, South America, and Africa have used coconut oil for everything from spiritual ceremonies to maintaining healthy skin to treating a multitude of illnesses. Here are just a few specific purposes that coconut oil has traditionally been used for:

- Hair conditioning
- Skin moisturizing
- Rubbing on babies to ensure good health and strong bones

- Heartburn
- Ulcers
- Reducing fevers
- Wound healing
- Maintaining a healthy heart
- Healthy bones
- Sunscreen
- Scar avoidance
- Cognitive function
- Adding delicious flavors to foods
- Crispy pastry crusts
- Source of nutrition
- Perfume
- Soap
- Base for cosmetics, both rudimentary and modern
- Treating skin conditions such as scabies, ringworm, and dermatitis
- Dental health
- Natural deodorant

Today, science backs up what natural healers already know: It's an antifungal, antibacterial, and antiviral as well as a source of *medium-chain triglycerides* (see Chapter 3). Researchers had given scientific credence to the wisdom gained by eons of trial and error.

Remember that all of these benefits were derived from coconut oil that was extracted naturally and gently, with no heat and no chemical processing that could damage the delicate antioxidants and other healthy ingredients. That makes a big difference, and you need to be aware of how your potential coconut oil was extracted before you buy it.

Coconut Oil Extraction Methods

The way that the oil is extracted from the coconut makes all the difference in the world to its healthfulness and flavor. As a matter of fact, it was the extraction and preparation method that earned coconut oil trouble way back in the 1960s. We will review the ways that coconut oil may be extracted and processed so you know what to look for when you're buying yours.

Before we get into the actual methods, it is important to note that the process involves either freshly dried meat or a combination of raw or dried meat and coconut milk. The former is called a *dry process* and the latter is called a *wet process*.

Pressing

For thousands of years, a cold-press method has been used that simply involved removing the meat from the mature nut, drying it, and then pressing the oil from the dried meat (or *copra*). The meat may be dried using the sun, fire, smoke, or a kiln. It's important that the coconut be mature so that the meat is thick and has absorbed all of the nutrient-rich, flavorful milk. After being pressed out of the meat, the milk and oil mix is allowed to settle for a day or two. During that time, known as the *fermentation time*, three layers will form: a top layer of cream and layers of protein and water.

Cold-pressing simply means that there is low or no heat used in the process, because heat can damage the nutrients and enzymes in the oil. Sometimes heat is used in the pressing method to extract more oil, but in general, a cold-pressing method, either manually or by machine, is preferred.

Aqueous Processing

The coconut meat is boiled in water until it gets soft and releases the oils. The coconut oil rises to the top and is collected. Boiling will destroy the antioxidants and many of the delicate nutrients found within the meat. Coconut oil derived from this process is not desirable for cooking or beauty products.

Centrifugal Extraction

This is a pretty simple method of extraction and can produce a high-quality coconut oil. The meat is placed into a machine that chops it up. The meat then goes through a screw press that takes the milk out. The dry meat finally goes into a high-speed centrifuge that spins the oil out of the meat so that it can be collected.

Expeller Extraction

This method can be either good or bad depending on whether or not chemicals and heat are used in the extraction process. The coconut meat is placed in a mechanical cylinder and pulverized and pressed into what's called a coconut cake. The heated coconut is then put into a barrel where a rod rotates and crushes the coconut, preparing it for extraction. Finally, the chemical *hexane* may be added to separate the cake from the oil, and the cake is then pressed to extract the oil. When hexane is used, the oil will need to be refined to remove the chemicals. This method causes quite a bit of frictional heat that may damage the oil.

Now that you know how the oil may be separated from the meat, let's talk a little bit about the different types of oil, what they taste like, and what they bring to the table nutritionally.

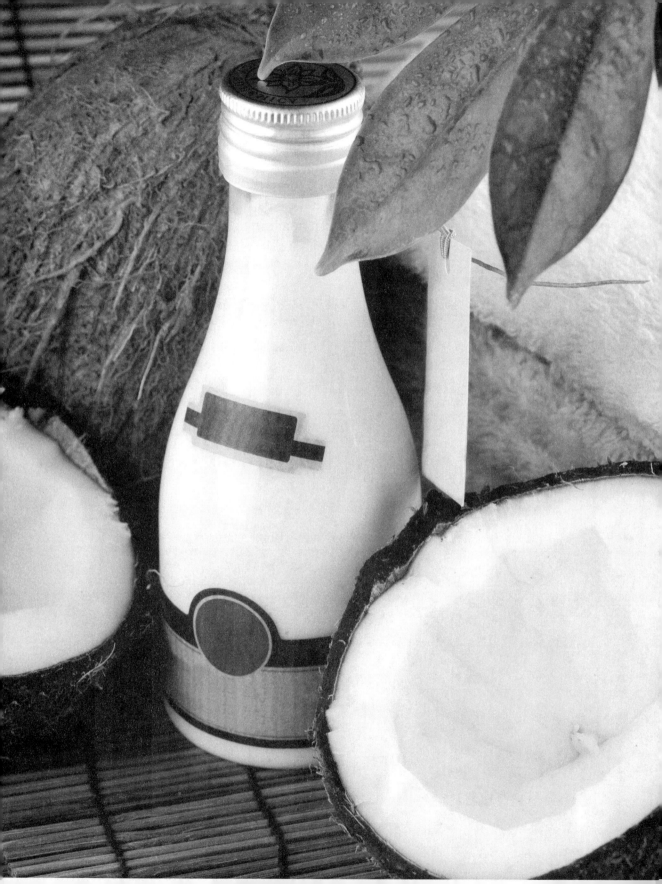

A SHOPPER'S GUIDE TO COCONUT OIL

In the land of coconuts, all oil is not made the same. Just as with other nut and vegetable oils, the quality of the product depends on the extraction process and whether or not the oil is refined. As with all produce, pesticides and other chemicals are a serious consideration that lends even more confusion to the buying process. There are several different forms of coconut oil adorning your grocer's shelf just waiting to be chosen, but how to choose?

Coconut Oil Buying Tip

When the term organic is applied to coconut oil, it only guarantees that the coconut palm or the oil itself wasn't treated with any fertilizers, pesticides, or solvents that aren't organic as defined by that country's certifying organization. It doesn't mean that the oil hasn't been refined or hydrogenated.

Refined Versus Unrefined Coconut Oil

Let's start with the two broadest categories, refined and unrefined, and then break it down further from there. There's not only a difference in the processing of refined and unrefined oil, but also a significant difference in taste.

Unrefined Coconut Oil

This type of oil is exactly what the name implies: It's left in the natural state after it's pressed. You may recognize this type better by its more common name: virgin coconut oil. Virgin oils are generally going to have a richer, nuttier flavor, and they will maintain the full nutritional value because they haven't been subjected to heat that can kill the delicate enzymes. Unrefined coconut oil has a shelf life of up to two years and a relatively high *smoke point* (the point at which taste and nutritional value degrade) of 350 degrees Fahrenheit.

Refined Coconut Oil

There are several reasons why coconut oil may be refined. First and foremost, refining removes impurities or chemicals that may have been used during the extraction process. The second reason for refining coconut oil is that it increases the smoke point so you can cook with it at higher temperatures without it burning and degrading. Finally, refined oils don't carry much coconut flavor, if any, so refining makes the coconut oil a more versatile product.

Refining isn't always bad; there are modern ways to do it using steam or diatomaceous earth (a soft sedimentary rock used as a filtration aid) to cleanse and purify the oil. Do your research before purchasing a refined coconut oil, so you know what you're getting!

Other Processes that Affect Nutritional Values

If you're using virgin or unrefined coconut oil, none of the following terms will be an issue, but if you want to use a refined oil for, say, frying foods without imparting a coconut flavor, then you need to be aware of the following processes in order to make an informed choice.

Refined, Bleached, and Deodorized (RBD)

Although this sounds like something that you'd do to your gym shoes after a long run, it's actually a common practice with fats and oils. Many oils go rancid quickly or are extracted with chemicals that can be harmful. Also, if the oil has gone rancid, a deodorizing process will be used to mask the smell. As you can probably guess, this process isn't exactly good for you or the oil.

Hydrogenated

In an attempt to increase the melting point, refined, saturated fats such as the ones found in coconut oil are combined with hydrogen particles to make them more saturated and thus more shelf stable. Hydrogenated coconut oil is used when you need a more solid product, such as when making cake icing. This process threw coconut oil under the bus with the rest of the unhealthy fats back in the 1960s because hydrogenation causes the formation of trans fats, the bad boys that cause heart disease and other potentially deadly disorders. Avoid hydrogenated fats, if you can.

Fractionated

Sometimes the medium-chain triglycerides (see Chapter 3) are separated out of coconut oil for specific purposes. Generally, fractionation is done for medical, cosmetic, dietary, or industrial needs. The triglycerides can be used as a nutrient in specific situations, so most likely you're not going to encounter this at the grocery store unless you're at a specialty athletic store.

Now you know what kind of coconut oil will suit your needs and which bad processes to avoid, but we still haven't discussed why coconut oil is such a great thing. Next, we'll talk about what makes it so good for you.

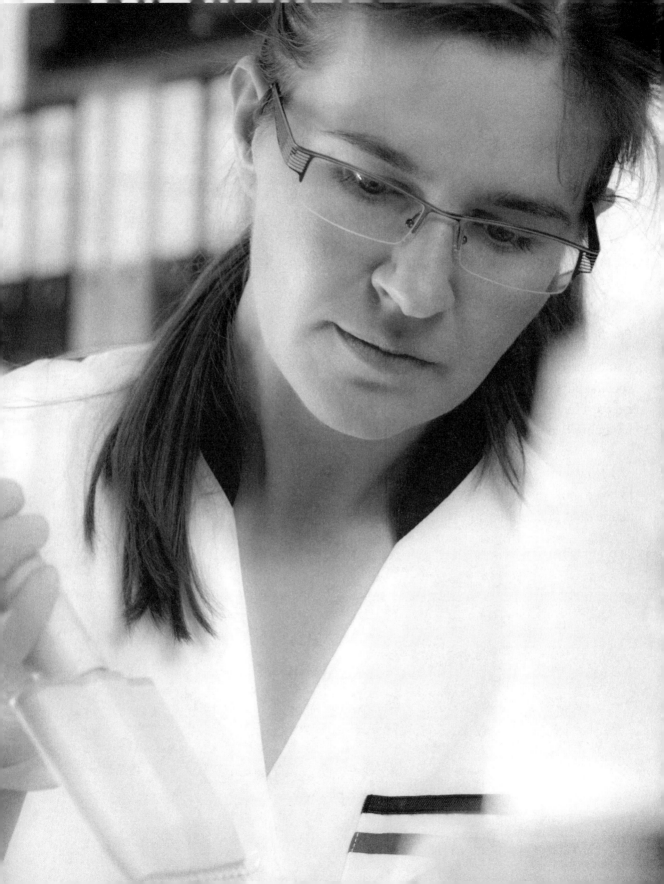

3

THE SCIENCE OF COCONUT OIL

In the late 1950s, when the health sciences started progressing in leaps and bounds, scientists noticed that saturated fats were linked to such lethal conditions as atherosclerosis, heart disease, and stroke. "Aha!" they said. "We've found the dietary link that can lead to a reduction in death and disability!" Indeed, they had, but they hadn't yet taken that research quite far enough to accurately define exactly what it was about saturated fats that caused those conditions.

As it turns out, all saturated fats are not created equal, and not only are some of them *not* bad for you, they're actually good for you. One of those healthy fats is the type found in coconut oil. The good fat isn't its only asset, either. Coconut oil is packed with nutrients, is an excellent healing agent, and kills a wide array of bad bugs that cause infection, illness, and disease.

Since the hardest part to understand is that the scientists messed up in the beginning, we're going to take a look at why the saturated fat in coconut oil is different from other "bad" types of saturated fats. This requires taking a step back to chemistry class for a couple of paragraphs, but it's important so you can understand the health benefits that we'll talk about later.

Debunking the Myth

The reason that coconut oil was lumped in with all of the other saturated fats to begin with is because the oil that was used in the original experiments was hydrogenated. We've already discussed the fact that hydrogenating oil causes trans fats to form, and it's those fats that wreak all of the havoc within your circulatory system. Pure coconut oil contains no trans fats and has actually been shown to do exactly the opposite of what it was originally accused of—it promotes heart and brain health and may accelerate the loss of unhealthy belly fat.

Why Is Coconut Oil's Fat Different?

Coconut oil has 116 calories and 14 grams of fat per tablespoon. Of those 14 grams of fat, 12 of them are saturated, but don't visualize your arteries clogging just yet! The saturated fat in coconut oil is made up of medium-chain triglycerides (MCT), not long-chain triglycerides (LCT)—the sort you'll find in many other forms of saturated fats. That difference is critical. Unlike LCTs that have to be broken down before they can be used, MCTs are broken down into medium-chain fatty acids that are absorbed relatively easily right in the digestive tract and are sent straight to your liver to be used for energy.

LCTs, on the other hand, are broken down in the digestive tract into long-chain fatty acids that require the use of pancreatic enzymes to break them into smaller, usable chunks. Then they're bundled together into fat packets called *lipoproteins* that are circulated throughout your body via your blood, where they leave fatty components in your different tissues. As they're used, they get smaller and are picked back up by your liver, and they are either broken down and used for energy or repackaged and sent back around again.

The condensed version of all of this? MCTs are largely converted to energy, while LCTs are often stored as fat.

Common Nutritional Uses of Coconut Oil

Because MCTs don't require excess energy from your body to absorb, use, or store them, they're often used to provide nutrition to patients who have problems absorbing or metabolizing nutrients or who use GI tubes for feeding. You'll also find coconut oil in baby formula and many sports drinks and foods because it is so easily absorbed and used. It will be listed as MCT because of the beating that coconut oil took from health professionals in the past.

Now that you understand the basic chemistry behind coconut oil's fat content, let's move on to other fascinating health benefits and uses.

SECTION TWO

Coconut Oil for Health

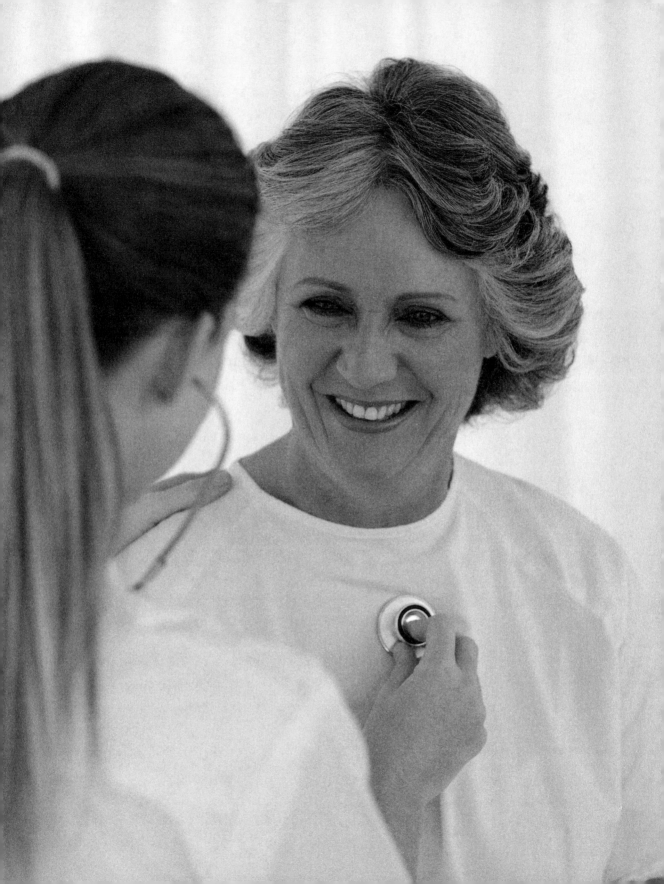

COCONUT OIL AS A DISEASE FIGHTER

In addition to being a ready source of energy, coconut oil has a wide array of other health benefits. Some of them, as discussed in Chapter 2, are related to healthy fats, while others are attributed to other aspects of the oil, such as the high amount of antioxidants it contains. The predominant fatty acid in coconut oil, *lauric acid*, is known to be beneficial in several different ways.

What Is Lauric Acid?

Lauric acid, a medium-chain fatty acid that is one of the components of triglycerides, is fairly uncommon except for in a few oils, including coconut oil. It accounts for about half of the fatty acid content of coconut oil and is one of the components that makes the oil so beneficial. It's thought to have microbial properties and has also been shown to increase high-density lipoprotein (HDL, or good cholesterol) levels in your blood. It also neutralizes with sodium hydroxide to form *sodium laurate* (aka soap).

How Does Coconut Oil Fight Disease and Boost Immunity?

Lauric acid is converted to *monolaurin*, a monoglyceride that's been shown to have antimicrobial, antiviral, and antifungal properties because it disrupts the fatty membranes of infectious agents, thus killing them. Your body uses monolaurin to fight bacterial infections as well as viruses and fungi caused by lipid-coated bugs, but because monolaurin is made from lauric acid, and saturated fats have become taboo, many people don't have enough monolaurin in their bodies to do any good.

Since coconut oil is nearly half lauric acid, it provides your body with what it needs to fight everything from the common cold to the big, bad bugs that cause such diseases as:

- Herpes
- Flu
- Measles
- Hepatitis
- Candida
- Ringworm
- Thrush
- Human immunodeficiency virus (HIV)

Lauric acid is also pretty much nontoxic and definitely nonaddictive, so if you compare it to modern drugs that are used to treat these conditions, you're certainly better off taking the natural route. Though there isn't any recommended daily intake of lauric acid, many health professionals suggest that three tablespoons of coconut oil per day will provide enough lauric acid to keep your immune system strong. This amount will also boost your metabolism and help keep your skin and hair healthy, too.

Coconut Oil Is an Anti-Inflammatory

Inflammation causes disease. That's not a supposition or a claim; it's a scientific fact. Inflammation in your body is responsible for a myriad of illnesses including heart disease, stroke, and even cancer. That's not even counting the obvious kinds of inflammation such as arthritis and the tissue swelling caused by hemorrhoids and soft tissue injuries. Studies have shown that coconut oil is indeed an anti-inflammatory and it also acts as a minor analgesic.

Healthy Bones, Teeth, Eyes, Skin, and Immune System

It's not a rumor and it's not hype—coconut oil really does help keep your entire body healthy because it aids in critical vitamin, mineral, and nutrient absorption. The medium-chain fatty acids that coconut oil is composed of are smaller in physical stature and are thus more easily absorbed. Also, there are some nutrients that are fat-soluble, which means that they need fat to be absorbed by the body. Since medium-chain triglycerides (MCTs) are smaller and more easily absorbed, they are great for helping your body absorb the fat-soluble goodies found in fruits and veggies. Just a few of these fat-soluble nutrients include:

- **Vitamin A**: There are two forms of vitamin A that your body uses: preformed vitamin A, also known as *retinoids* and provitamin-A (aka carotenoids). Retinoids are found in animal products such as fish, meat, and dairy, while carotenoids are from vegetable sources.

   Vitamin A is necessary for good eye health and is actually a huge factor in preventing eye disorders such as macular degeneration and cataracts. It's also known to help protect against severe measles, physical signs of aging, and cancer. In fact, vitamin A plays a critical role in the health of all major organs and systems, partly because of its powerful antioxidant powers and partly because it plays a tremendous role in cell communication and differentiation.

- **Vitamin D**: Most people get all the vitamin D they need from the sun, but many cereals and milk are supplemented with it, too. It helps your body absorb calcium, and people who don't get enough vitamin D are at risk of developing thin, porous, brittle bones, a condition known as *rickets* in kids and *osteomalacia* in adults. Insufficient calcium is also linked to osteoporosis. Vitamin D also helps carry messages from your brain to the rest of your body, and your immune system needs it to fight off bacterial and viral diseases.

- **Vitamin E**: You're exposed to free radicals just about everywhere. Free radicals are naturally occurring but highly reactive molecules. They're in the air that you breathe, just about everything that you touch, the food you eat, and even in the sun. Your body actually makes a certain amount of free radicals in order to rid your body of toxins, but when you have too many, they cause serious damage because they create oxidation in healthy cells. This can lead to physical signs of aging as well as cancer, brain deterioration, and general havoc throughout your body. Vitamin E is a powerful antioxidant that also enhances the use of other antioxidants.

   Vitamin E also plays a critical role in helping your immune system fight disease, and it helps keep your circulatory system healthy by widening your vessels and preventing clots from forming. Finally, vitamin E helps your cells to communicate. Alas, it requires fat to be absorbed.

- **Vitamin K**: This is yet another nutrient that's critical to numerous vital bodily functions including clotting, bone health, and prevention of calcification in your tissues that can cause atherosclerosis, heart disease, vascular disease, Alzheimer's disease, and stroke. Vitamin K is a powerful antioxidant that protects your cells from oxidation, and it is also an anti-inflammatory that lowers *interleukin-6*, an inflammatory marker linked to diseases such as cancer. Finally, vitamin K is essential for the formation of *sphingolipids* (fats) that form the outer wrapping of nerves, called the *myelin sheath*.

None of these vitamins can be absorbed by your body without fatty acids, and medium-chain fatty acids are arguably the best for the job. You should know, however, that too much of a good thing in this case is a bad thing. Because fat-soluble vitamins are stored, you can become toxic if you consume extreme amounts of them.

Though your body needs these vitamins, there's generally not a need to supplement as long as you're healthy and eat a well-balanced diet. This includes healthy fatty acids such as the ones found in coconut oil so that your body can absorb the vitamins. As with all things, moderation is key. You need to eat healthy fats when you consume fat-soluble nutrients, but that means using coconut oil as a component of your salad dressing or to sauté your fish. You don't need to drink a glass of it!

Coconut Oil and Alzheimer's Disease

In addition to shuttling vital nutrients to your brain, studies show that MCT administered to people with mild cognitive impairment or Alzheimer's disease showed almost immediate increases in *ketone bodies* that are associated with measurable levels of improved cognitive function in people with mild to moderate cognitive impairment.

Coconut Oil and Heart Disease

Coconut oil helps keep your heart healthy in a couple of different ways. We've just reviewed how it helps with the absorption of heart-healthy fat-soluble vitamins, but it also acts as an antioxidant in its own right, thus protecting your cells from oxidation and keeping your arteries free from plaque buildup. Furthermore, MCTs raise the levels of "good" HDL cholesterol as well as "bad" LDL cholesterol. It's an imbalance in the two that's now known to cause problems.

As long as there's a healthy balance, levels stay in a healthy range. Long-chain triglycerides raise only the bad cholesterol and thus give saturated fats their bad reputation.

Coconut Oil Is an Antimicrobial

Again, this is fact, not supposition. Research shows that coconut oil, both digested and applied topically, kills bacteria, viruses, fungi, and other bad bugs. People use it to promote dental health by swishing it around in much the same fashion as mouthwash. Swishing coconut oil, a process also referred to as *oil pulling*, is thought to act as a whole-body detoxifier. Coconut oil treated with enzymes to mimic digestion was shown to inhibit *Streptococcus*, the bacteria known to cause dental plaque. Throughout history it's also been a valuable component of poultices and salves because of its germ-fighting ability.

Coconut Health Fact

In times of war or emergency, coconut water can be used in place of IV blood plasma because it is sterile, is nutrient rich, and has the exact same pH as human blood.

If we were to go into detail about every single health benefit of coconut oil, we'd be here for a long time; however, this chapter presented some of the top reasons. There is one more health area where coconut oil really shines, and we'd like to touch on it before moving ahead to the beauty benefits. That area is stress and anti-aging. Since coconut oil has several beauty as well as health applications in this area, it merits its own chapter.

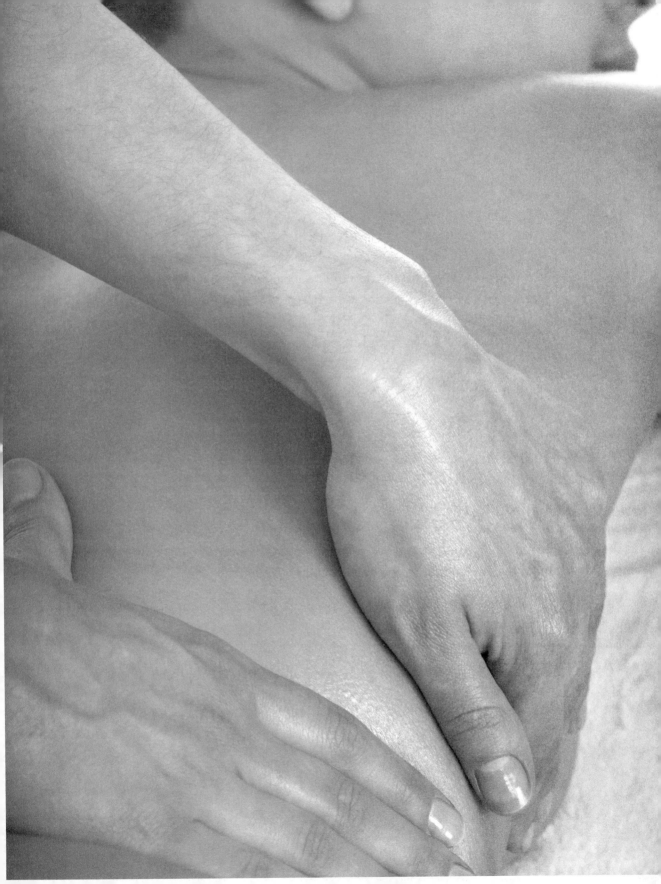

COCONUT OIL FOR STRESS RELIEF AND ANTI-AGING

If there was a single product that could get rid of dry skin, protect you from the sun, make you look younger, and help you relax, you'd rush straight out and buy it, wouldn't you? Well, as you've probably already guessed, we're talking about coconut oil. We've spent several chapters talking about the many benefits that coconut oil has when you eat it, so now we're going to talk about how much it can help you by wearing it.

Coconut Oil and Anti-Aging

The anti-aging market is a multi-billion-dollar global industry, mostly because nobody wants to be old and sick. There are products that are designed with all sorts of man-made chemicals and "natural" ingredients that are supposedly formulated just to eliminate the external signs of aging. As a matter of fact, there are some truly effective ingredients out there, but they're often lost among the snake oils. One ingredient that wasn't used much until recently is coconut oil.

That would be partly because, just as in nutrition circles, fats have been ostracized in the world of skin care. They supposedly cause everything from acne to cancer and, again, as in the world of nutrients, fats have all been lumped together, the good with the bad. It's true that some oils clog your pores, dry you out, cause oxidation, and spread bacteria, but coconut oil isn't one of them. As a matter of fact, coconut oil does just the opposite.

Antioxidants

Virgin coconut oil is rich in antioxidants called *phytonutrients* that protect your skin from the damaging effects of the sun's rays and free radicals. You're exposed to these unstable molecules just by existing, and if left unchecked, they will cause ashy skin, wrinkles, thinning skin, and age spots. Free radicals have also been linked to skin cancer, so the antioxidants in coconut oil not only keep you looking young, they can also save your life!

Healing Agents

We've already discussed the fact that coconut oil has antibacterial, antiviral, and antimicrobial properties, and this is perfect if you're trying to maintain or achieve healthy skin. Many people believe that acne is caused by clogged pores, but it's actually bacteria that cause the problem. Coconut oil can help improve or even cure your acne because it kills harmful bacteria. It can also help with such problems as fungal infections that make your skin itchy, red, or scaly. It also helps to slough off dead skin cells so that fresh, glowing skin can grow underneath.

Moisturizing

Most of the products on the market today have water or mineral oil as primary ingredients. Water is great, but it plumps your skin up for a while before it evaporates, and the wrinkles just come back. Mineral oil is typically refined and may contain free radicals and other ingredients that damage your skin and make you look older.

This is where the medium-chain fatty acids come back into play. Because the molecules are smaller than those that make up other oils (even the ones that could potentially be good for you) it can penetrate your skin more easily so that its moisture and those amazing antioxidants can get in there and fight free radicals, bacteria, and dry skin where it really matters—inside your tissues.

Nutrient Delivery

Remember how medium-chain fatty acids help with nutrient absorption? It does the same thing with your skin. Since they're small enough to penetrate your skin, they can take healing, anti-aging nutrients such as vitamins A and E with it so that your skin can heal from the inside. It's even possible that coconut oil can help carry *collagen*, the protein that forms the tissues that hold your skin firmly in place. Wrinkles, saggy skin, and age spots will improve, and you'll look younger naturally.

Sunscreen

If you look at Pacific Islanders, they have beautiful, bronze skin without cancer or blemish, and that's due in large part to their use of coconuts both internally and topically. Coconut oil is shown to protect you from damaging UVA and UVB rays by blocking up to 70 percent of those rays from ever touching your skin. Since damage from sun rays is a huge contributor to old-looking skin, this is a huge part of looking younger.

Stress Relief

Massage is used to relieve stress that can cause illness and disease. It improves circulation and helps stimulate healing in your muscles and soft tissues. Used for centuries to heal and promote good health, massage is an integral part of natural medicine. Using coconut oil as a massage oil has several advantages over other oils. Here are some of them:

- The natural antibacterial agents in coconut oil keep it from going rancid or spreading germs over your body.

- The ability to deeply penetrate the skin moisturizes and softens your skin.

- The antioxidants help keep your skin young and healthy.

- It can help carry healing herbs, essential oils, and extracts into your skin so that you can target specific problems.

- It smells fantastic without being overwhelming.

- The high fat content keeps it from getting sticky during the massage.

Whether you'd like to use coconut oil for anti-aging, massage therapy, or a combination thereof, there are many different ways to use it. You can either use it by itself or you can incorporate other ingredients with it. For instance, vitamin A (aka retinol) is known for its wrinkle-reducing powers, so you can mix a little vitamin A into your coconut oil. This is just an example—the options are virtually unlimited.

Over the next several chapters, we're going to discuss more beauty benefits of coconut oil and also share some great recipes, including ones for anti-aging products and massage oils.

Coconut Oil for Beauty

- **Chapter 6:** Coconut Oil for Your Hair

- **Chapter 7:** Coconut Oil for Your Skin

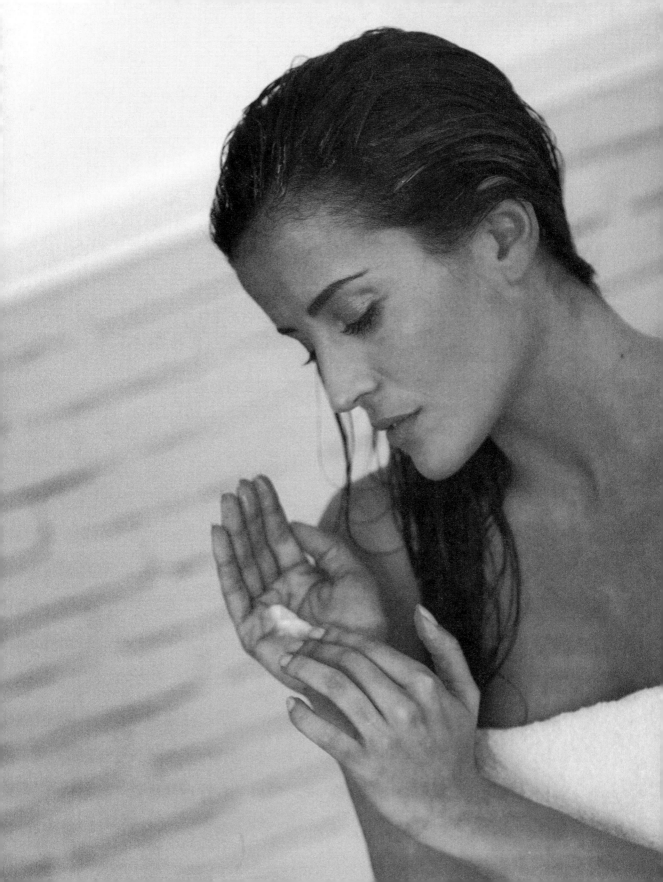

$$\bigcirc 6$$

COCONUT OIL FOR YOUR HAIR

For millennia, people have used coconut oil to keep hair hydrated and beautiful, and recently, it's become a popular ingredient in many hair care products. And why not? It smells good, it's natural, and it works. As a matter of fact, scientific studies prove that coconut oil, unlike most other products, actually penetrates the hair shaft. This is due in large part to the structural composition of the oil. We've already discussed the smaller composition of coconut oil compared to other oils, and it's that smaller molecular size that allows it to get into the shaft.

Why Most Hair Products Don't Work

The core of your hair is covered in protective plates called *cuticles*. When your hair shaft or cuticles become damaged from heat, styling products, or environmental pollutants, your hair starts to look frizzy, limp, and dull. Unfortunately, the first ingredients in most products are water and refined vegetable oils such as mineral oil or even hydrogenated vegetable oil.

The water is fine, but it doesn't contribute to the health of your hair. The oils, on the other hand, can actually do further damage. Once oil is refined, it loses the antioxidants that protect it from oxidizing so that it becomes a source of free radicals. Instead of moisturizing and protecting your hair, it's actually harming it. Virgin coconut oil is rich in antioxidants and protects and nourishes your hair.

Even if the oil is good, chances are good that it's not going to penetrate your hair shaft, because the molecules are too big. As a result, the product just sits on the outside of your hair. This may make your hair feel good, and even look good as long as the product is on your hair, but as soon as you wash it off, your hair is still brittle and unhealthy. The medium-chain triglycerides (MCTs) found in coconut oil slip right to the cortex of your hair where they can work to restore healthy resilience.

Dandruff

Flakey, itchy, and embarrassing, dandruff is a problem for many people. If you're one of them, you know how difficult it is to find an effective treatment. Some of the ingredients that you'll find in dandruff shampoos include ketoconazole, zinc pyrithione, and selenium sulfide, all of which are fungicides. These are used because, contrary to popular belief, dandruff isn't caused by dry skin; it's caused by a fungus similar to the one that causes yeast infections. It can also be caused by an overly oily scalp.

A coconut oil scalp treatment is great for both causes. If you recall, coconut oil has antifungal properties and helps old skin cells to slough off. The massaging action that you'll be using to apply it will help loosen the layers of buildup and promote a healthy level of oil production, which is the result of improved circulation under your scalp.

Regardless of whether you choose to use basic coconut oil or to go for one of the fancier infused mixes, warm your treatment up a bit prior to using it, especially considering that it's in a semisolid state at room temperature. Don't heat it too much, though. Just make it a bit warm so that it soothes your scalp. After you rub it in, put a shower cap on and let it sit for a few minutes. You'll need only a couple of tablespoons to treat your entire scalp.

Finally, remember to massage your scalp with the tips of your fingers instead of using your fingernails. You don't want to run the risk of damaging your scalp by scratching, which can cause infections and make your dandruff worse.

Head Lice

If you have schoolkids, you've probably learned to cringe when you hear these dreaded words. Once you get them, it seems like they're nearly impossible to get rid of. They infest your hair first and then the rest of your house. Once you get them, you have to treat for them several times to get rid of them because they lay eggs that hatch quickly and then *they* lay more eggs. Standard treatments involve hazardous chemicals that have some terrifying side effects. For example:

- **Permethrin:** This insecticide kills lice by acting as a neurotoxin. It interrupts communication between nerve cells and causes seizures, paralysis, and then death. Permethrin is often used in flea treatments for dogs but is extremely toxic to cats because they can't metabolize the poison fast enough. Side effects for people include vomiting, pneumonia, muscle paralysis, respiratory failure, and asthma.

- **Carbaryl:** This insecticide is in the carbarnate family of pesticides and also acts on the central nervous system. Side effects include stomach cramps, nausea, vomiting, diarrhea, drooling, blurred vision, poor coordination, and even seizures.

Remember that you're not just putting this on your hair; you're putting it on your scalp, too. This means that it's being absorbed into your bloodstream or into your child's bloodstream. Another consideration is that research shows that lice are building resistance to these toxins, so you may be risking these awful side effects without even killing the bugs. The inactive ingredients of head lice shampoos typically include alcohol and other chemicals that dry your hair out and make it susceptible to damage.

So what's the best course of action if you want a safe, effective way to kill head lice? Coconut oil! Used alone, it's extremely effective, but when you pair it with other natural ingredients or herbals, studies show that it's every bit as effective as chemical pesticides. The two most common partner ingredients include apple cider vinegar and anise. The vinegar and anise help dissolve the glue that holds the eggs onto your hair shaft. Check the following recipes section to find out how to treat head lice.

Healthy Hair

So with all of the conflicting information out there, how can you tell exactly what are the best ways to use coconut oil for increasing the health of your hair without getting a greasy look? The answer is you can use it in numerous ways, including as a finishing hair serum, as long as you use it sparingly. Research proves that when used regularly, especially as a prewash such as a hot-oil-style treatment, coconut oil helps your hair maintain proteins that keep it healthy. Some great ways to incorporate coconut oil into your hair care routine include:

- Hot-oil treatment
- Shampoo

- Conditioner
- Leave-in conditioner
- Finishing serum

There are some great recipes in the following section, but don't be afraid to get creative. If you like the smell of jasmine or lime, incorporate those into your recipes. Research a bit first just to make sure that it's safe to use for whatever you want to use it for.

Melting Coconut Oil

Virgin coconut oil melts at 76 degrees Fahrenheit, so not much is needed to melt it. You can place the coconut oil container in a bowl of hot water or melt what you need in a small pan over low heat. Avoid microwaving, if possible. Don't use melted coconut oil in the recipes unless instructed to.

Coconut Oil Hair Care Recipes

Coconut oil has a fairly long shelf life—up to two years or more depending upon how it's stored, so it's OK to make this stuff in batches as long as the other ingredients are stable as well.

Coconut Oil Head Lice Treatment

There are numerous old wives' tales about things that can kill lice, and there is some credence to many of them. Research shows that pennyroyal, marjoram, tea tree oil, lavender, eucalyptus, anise, ylang-ylang, and rosemary effectively kill head lice. Coconut oil by itself isn't nearly as effective without the addition of some of these other ingredients.

- ½ cup virgin coconut oil, melted
- 8 drops lavender oil
- 8 drops ylang-ylang oil
- ½ cup apple cider vinegar

In a glass bowl, mix together coconut oil, lavender oil, and ylang-ylang oil, and set aside.

Apply the vinegar to your hair to saturate it. Then allow to air dry. The vinegar dissolves the glue that holds the eggs to the hair shaft so that the eggs will be easy to comb out.

When your hair is dry, apply the coconut oil mixture, making sure that you get your scalp coated.

Put a shower cap on and leave on for at least 2 hours.

Using a nit comb, remove all dead lice and eggs from scalp and hair. Wash out with shampoo. Repeat every 3 days, 3 times a day.

Yields 1 application.

Coconut Oil Hot-Oil Treatment

Both jojoba and lavender are excellent for your hair, and of course, the coconut oil adds moisture and helps your hair retain the proteins that keep it lush and beautiful.

- ¼ cup virgin coconut oil, melted
- 8 drops jojoba oil
- 8 drops lavender oil

Mix all ingredients together in a glass bowl and apply to slightly damp hair, working your way from the roots to the ends.

Warm your hair with a hair dryer and cover it with a shower cap. Leave on for up to 1 hour, and then wash as usual. You'll probably need to wash your hair at least twice to clean the oils from your hair.

Yields 1 treatment.

Coconut Oil After-Styling Serum

This serum smells fabulous and will help keep your hair sleek and shiny. Be extremely careful though, because it takes only a tiny amount to do the trick. Otherwise, you'll look greasy instead of chic! Make up a batch and put it in a little squeeze bottle.

- 1 tablespoon virgin coconut oil
- 6 drops pineapple oil

Mix the coconut oil and pineapple oil together in a squeeze bottle and shake. Or if you're not using a squeeze bottle, just mix them together well.

Put 2 to 3 drops on your palm and rub your hands together. Run your hands over your hair, smoothing as you go.

Yields about 1 month's worth of serum.

Coconut Basic Shampoo

This is great if you just want to get your hair clean without adding any herbs or other nonnecessities to it. The coconut oil will help preserve the protein, and the baking soda acts as a gentle scrub for your scalp.

- 2 ounces liquid castile soap
- 4 ounces distilled water
- 1 teaspoon virgin coconut oil
- 2 tablespoons aloe vera gel
- 2 tablespoons baking soda

Add all ingredients to a small bowl and stir well.

Store in a shampoo bottle and use just like you'd use any other shampoo, but you'll most likely need less. Although it may look watery, it's really not. It lathers up nicely with just a little bit. If you'd like to skip the castile soap altogether, just replace it with water.

Yields about 10 liquid ounces.

Coconut Herbal Shampoo

This basic shampoo is easy to mix up. If you really want to be a chemist, there are many different "scratch" soap recipes out there, but this one is much simpler. Be careful using essential oils, because some of them will alter your hair color; for instance, chamomile will have a mild lightening effect, so if you have dark hair, you may want to avoid that. If you have dandruff, add a little tea tree oil to the mix.

- 2 teaspoons dried rose petals
- 1 teaspoon dried marshmallow root
- 2 teaspoons dried violet leaf
- 10 ounces distilled water
- 4 ounces liquid castile soap
- ¼ teaspoon virgin coconut oil
- ¼ teaspoon jojoba oil
- 3 tablespoons aloe vera gel
- 25 drops lavender oil
- 5 to 10 drops tea tree oil for dandruff, if necessary

Add the rose petals, marshmallow root, and violet leaf to a jar or small glass bowl.

Bring the distilled water to a boil and pour over the dried herbs. Allow them to steep until the mix is cool.

Strain the herbs out and discard. Pour the herbed water into a shampoo bottle or whatever container you wish to use.

Add the castile soap to the bottle. Then add the coconut oil and jojoba oil.

Add the aloe vera and the lavender oil and shake to combine. Add the tea tree oil if desired. You'll need to shake it each time that you use it because it will separate. Use just as you'd use regular shampoo.

Yields about 1 month's worth of shampoo depending on how long your hair is.

Easy Coconut Leave-in Conditioner

This is about as simple as it gets, but your hair will reap the benefits for days after you use this conditioner. The vitamin E provides extra antioxidant power that, when combined with the coconut oil's permeability, makes for a great-smelling, healthy conditioner with no harsh chemicals or other ingredients that will weigh your hair down or cause damage.

- 2 tablespoons virgin coconut oil
- 4 liquid vitamin E capsules
- 5 drops of your favorite essential oil

Put the coconut oil in a small bowl. Poke a hole in the vitamin E capsules and squeeze them into the coconut oil.

Add your favorite essential oil. (Pineapple and mango are both great if you like the tropical smell.)

Mix them all together and add to a small bottle. Shake well before each use.

To use, place two to three drops on your palm and rub your hands together. Then run your hands through damp hair, concentrating on the hair shafts. It takes only a tiny amount or else your hair will look greasy. Used correctly, your hair will be smooth and shiny, and the longer you use this, the healthier your hair will become.

Yields about 1 month's worth of product.

Deep-Penetrating Coconut Oil Scalp Treatment

As you might imagine, many hair problems originate with poor scalp health. This soothing treatment helps stimulate healthy hair by removing conditioner and hair-gel buildup, repairing dry and damaged skin, and alleviating dandruff. Repeat this treatment once a month or as often as desired for exquisite-looking hair.

- 6 tablespoons virgin coconut oil
- 4 to 6 drops tea tree oil
- 4 to 6 drops rosemary oil

Place all ingredients in a small glass bowl and mix well. For best results, place the bowl in a shallow pan of warm water to soften.

Rub a generous amount of the treatment onto your scalp and massage it in for several minutes.

Cover your head with a shower cap or towel, and rinse the treatment out after 30 minutes.

Note that some people's skin is sensitive to tea tree oil. If you have this sensitivity, use only 2 to 3 drops and rinse out the treatment after 15 to 20 minutes.

Yields about 3 treatments.

Now that you have some great recipes for your hair, let's move on and talk a little more about how fabulous coconut oil is for your skin.

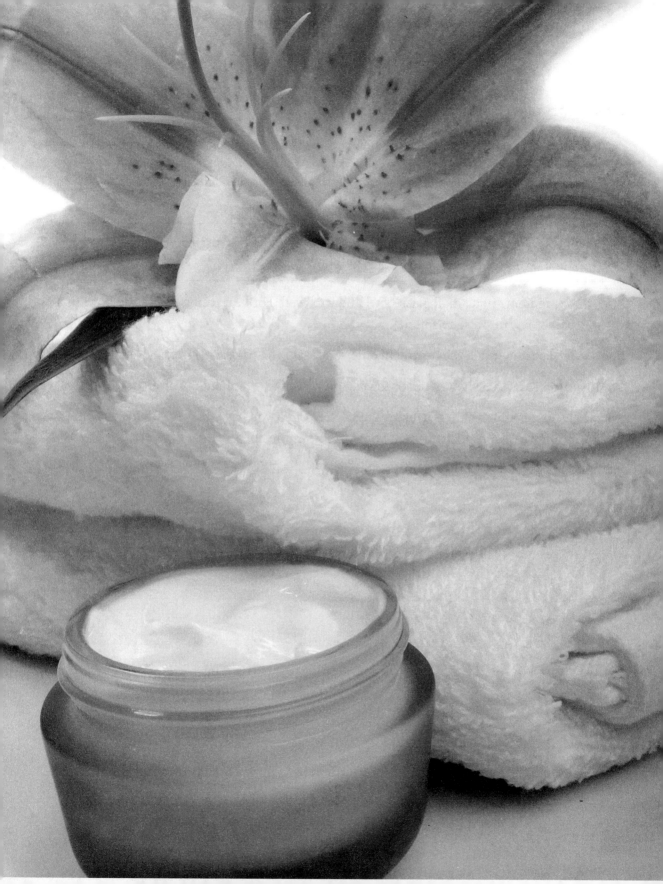

(7)

COCONUT OIL FOR YOUR SKIN

We already know that people have been slathering on the coconut oil for hundreds of years without the need for any scientific tests or proof. They just used it because it worked. But now research is piling up in just about every area of skin care to support the use of this luscious-smelling concoction. It's great for everything from simple moisturization to healing scars and helping reduce the appearance of wrinkles. And you can thank those magical medium-chain triglycerides (MCTs) that we've been discussing. In this chapter, you're going to learn some useful ways to incorporate coconut oil into your beauty routine so that you can see for yourself how incredible your skin can feel again!

Long-Lasting Moisture

One of the biggest problems many people have with commercial lotions is that the products work really well for an hour or two but then seem to simply stop, leaving skin just as dry (or drier) and flakey as it was before. There are a couple of reasons why this is so. First, the primary ingredient in most lotions is water. This is great, except that water evaporates, and without a medium to hold it in your skin, it won't be there for long, especially in a dry environment. Coconut oil's MCTs are a great transporter for water since they're small enough to penetrate your skin.

Another reason why your skin may feel drier after your lotion absorbs (or evaporates, as the case may be) is because it contains alcohol in one form or another. Certain forms of alcohol are used by auto mechanics to remove water from parts, so if alcohol is a dehydrator for cars, what do you think it's doing to your skin? There are also innumerable other chemicals used in moisturizers as binding agents and preservatives that can cause dryness, allergic reactions, and even long-term problems such as cancer.

Remember that your skin is your largest organ. It's porous and absorbs what you put on it, at least in part. Parabens, alcohols, and hydrogenated oils that contain free radicals are all common ingredients that you routinely slather onto your outer sponge. These may then be absorbed into your bloodstream. In essence, your skin "eats" some of what it comes into contact with, so should you really put anything on your skin that you wouldn't put in your mouth?

Protection from Bacteria, Viruses, and Fungi

Your body's first and most effective defense against infectious organisms is your skin; particularly the acidic layer of oil (aka sebum) that coats your skin. Our skin is slightly acidic (with a pH of around 5 to 5.5), creating an environment in which good bacteria can exist and go about their business but bad bugs can't. Some bacteria, in fact, are essential to good health. For example, there's at least one type that eats sebum (like anything else, too much of anything—in this case, sebum—is not good for your skin), breaking down the MCT in the process and leaving behind medium-chain fatty acids. MCTs aren't microbial, but once those fatty acids are released, they become powerful antimicrobials that combine with the slightly acidic environment on your skin to protect you from all sorts of different illnesses caused by "bad" bacteria, fungi, and viruses.

The layer of sebum on your skin consists of about 60 percent medium-chain fatty acids, but when you bathe, you wash much of that away, leaving your skin vulnerable. If you have a cut or some dry, cracked skin without the protective layer of sebum, it's like leaving the barn door open for anything that wants to enter. By applying coconut oil, you speed up the process of reestablishing the natural barrier.

Now that you know coconut oil protects you from disease while it's making you soft and young-looking, doesn't it make sense to use it after bathing?

Psoriasis and Other Skin Conditions

Despite what many people think, conditions such as psoriasis are not caused by a lack of moisture or fungi. It's caused by your body's inflammatory response. Basically, your body is having an allergic reaction to itself. And since coconut oil is an anti-inflammatory, it's great for these conditions. People seem to see a reduction in many different disorders (not just those caused by immune responses) after either applying coconut oil topically or eating it. Just a few of these disorders include:

- Psoriasis
- Eczema
- Keratosis pilaris
- Acne
- Seborrheic eczema
- Cold sores
- Cutaneous candidiasis

There are also some great uses for coconut oil for people who don't have specific skin conditions. Since it's an antimicrobial that moisturizes, soothes, and forms a protective lipid barrier wherever you apply it, think about substituting it for your everyday cosmetics including:

- Lip gloss
- Sunscreen
- Callus remover
- Body scrub
- Anti-aging cream
- Deodorant
- Toothpaste
- Soap

Simply substituting plain virgin coconut oil for many of these will work wonderfully, but the rest of this chapter features recipes that combine the power of other ingredients to blend with the coconut oil to make a truly superior product that is both effective and free of harmful chemicals.

Just a note: Your body is used to producing sweat and excess oil in response to chemicals and soap that you use. It's going to take your body time to adjust to being back to a natural state, so you may notice some excess sweating or oilier hair or skin for up to two months after you stop using chemicals that strip natural oils from your body. This is normal, so push through it. Your skin and hair will thank you!

Tropical Healing Massage Oil

Both coconut oil and sweet almond oil are nice, light oils that are easily absorbed. Jojoba is a bit waxier, so it gives the oil a little bit of drag that helps when you're doing deep-tissue massage. All have healing and restorative properties, and when you add the rosehip and ylang-ylang oils, tired, damaged skin is sure to feel better in no time. The vanilla and orange oils make it smell wonderful, too.

- 2 ounces virgin coconut oil
- 2 ounces sweet almond oil
- 2 ounces jojoba oil
- 1½ ounces rosehip oil
- 10 drops orange oil
- 10 drops vanilla oil
- 10 drops ylang-ylang oil

Blend all ingredients together and store in a glass bottle at room temperature. Don't use plastics, because you run the risk of phthalates from the plastic leeching into your oil. Warm the concoction up in the palm of your hand a bit before using to avoid a cold jolt when it hits your skin. You could also use this as a bath oil if you'd like.

Yields about 8 ounces.

Relaxation Massage Oil

Massage is as much a sensory experience as it is a hands-on, physical therapy session. The combination of essential oils and deep massage techniques using this oil will erase your tension and leave you relaxed and ready to rest.

- 2 ounces virgin coconut oil
- 2 ounces jojoba oil
- 2 ounces sweet almond oil
- 15 drops ylang-ylang oil
- 15 drops sandalwood oil

Combine all ingredients and store in a glass bottle. The shelf life for these ingredients is particularly long, especially if you store the concoction at room temperature. Warm the oil up in the palm or your hand before applying. It is also great as a bath oil.

Yields about 6 ounces.

Basic Healing Coconut Moisturizer

One of the best things about coconut oil is its ability to penetrate the skin; without that, none of the other uses would be as effective. Vitamin E is a healing restorative that is excellent for chapped skin and even fresh scars and wounds, but it needs fatty acids to unlock its lipid barrier so it can work. Coconut oil's medium-chain fatty acids make it a great transporter, since it both dissolves the vitamin E for use and helps it penetrate the skin where it can work.

- 6 liquid vitamin E capsules
- ½ cup virgin coconut oil

In a small glass bowl, poke a hole in the vitamin E capsules and squeeze them into the coconut oil. Stir to combine and slather onto your skin after you shower or whenever you're feeling a little dry.

This is great for dry spots too and is even useful for softening calluses. If you'd like to use it for calluses, simply slather on, cover, and leave on for a few hours or overnight. Wipe off the excess and that callus will be soft enough to slough off with your pedicure file.

Yields ½ cup moisturizer.

Soothing, Fragrant, Cherry-Vanilla Coconut Moisturizer

By adding vitamins and essential oils to your basic moisturizer, you can turn a utilitarian cream into a luxuriously soothing moisturizer that makes an amazing gift when packaged in a pretty jar . . . if you want to share it! Feel free to get creative with your oils to create a sensory experience that's pleasing to you.

- 1 cup virgin coconut oil
- ¼ cup jojoba oil
- 6 liquid vitamin E capsules
- 15 drops cherry essential oil
- 15 drops vanilla essential oil

Put the coconut oil and jojoba oil in a small bowl.

Poke a hole in each vitamin E capsule and squeeze it into the coconut oil. Discard the empty capsules.

Add the essential oils and stir until all of the ingredients are combined. Store in a glass jar at room temperature. Just rub the moisturizer on after your shower or whenever you feel dry.

Yields about 1¼ cups.

Anti-Aging Super Night Cream

This cream is packed with antioxidants, natural healing agents, and skin protectants that will help you fight wrinkles, age spots, and other signs of aging. Since coconut oil penetrates so easily and dissolves fat-soluble vitamins, it can help carry the nutrients deep within your skin so they can rebuild and repair from within. Vitamin A degrades in sunlight, so in order to get the full benefits, only use this at night.

- 2 tablespoons virgin coconut oil
- 2 tablespoons cherry kernel oil
- 1 tablespoon jojoba oil
- 6 liquid vitamin E capsules
- 6 liquid vitamin A capsules
- 5 drops lavender oil
- 5 drops frankincense oil

Add coconut, cherry kernel, and jojoba oils to a small bowl. Poke each vitamin E and vitamin A capsule and squeeze into the oils, discarding the empty capsules.

Add the lavender and frankincense oils, and then stir until all of the ingredients are thoroughly combined. Store in a dark-colored glass bottle or jar.

Apply at night before going to bed. It won't take much, so this amount will last you for quite a while. If you're sensitive to scents, you can leave out the lavender and frankincense oils and still have an incredible anti-aging concoction.

Yields about ¼ cup.

Lemon Zest and Brown Sugar Scrub

This is a great scrub to use on your face because unlike other facial scrubs, the brown sugar and lemon zest won't tear your skin when you use it. Always be gentle when using anything containing abrasive materials on your face because you can cause microscopic tears that let in acne-causing germs or bacteria. The citric acid in the lemon zest works with the coconut oil to slough off those dead skin cells so that your face glows.

- 1 tablespoon virgin or refined coconut oil
- 1 teaspoon brown sugar
- 1 teaspoon fresh lemon zest

In a small bowl, mix all three ingredients together. Place in a makeup pot and store any leftovers at room temperature for up to a week.

To use, pull your hair back and massage a small amount of the scrub gently onto your face, using only as much as you need to cover your face. Once you feel the coconut oil starting to absorb, rinse with lukewarm water until the sugar and lemon zest are gone and your face feels clean. Your skin will feel super-soft after using this scrub.

Yields almost 2 tablespoons of scrub.

Mango Mania Coconut Oil Lip Balm

You don't actually need anything else besides the coconut oil to make an effective gloss that hydrates your lips and helps protect them from the sun, but adding other ingredients can help mix it up and add new flavors and textures. Just make sure that anything you add to your lip balm is edible!

- 1 teaspoon virgin coconut oil
- 1 teaspoon organic mango butter, not melted
- 1 drop food-grade cherry flavoring oil

In a small dish, combine all three ingredients. Place in a reusable lip-balm pot or a small glass container.

Use the tip of your finger to apply a small amount to your lips. Mango butter has no flavor, so this is going to taste mostly cherry with a hint of coconut. If you'd like other flavors, just substitute other food-grade oils for the cherry. Make sure that they're oil soluble so they'll mix with the coconut oil and mango butter.

Yields 2 teaspoons lip balm.

All-Natural Deodorant

Commercial deodorants generally contain some form of aluminum, which has been linked to various illnesses, including cancer. It also often contains parabens and chemicals that can be harmful to your body. Body odor is caused by bacteria, and coconut oil, as we know, is a natural antibacterial. Feel free to choose your own essential oils, or just leave them out. Sometimes they can be irritating, so use a small bit in a practice batch before making a huge batch with it.

- ½ cup virgin or naturally refined coconut oil
- ¼ cup arrowroot powder (or cornstarch)
- ¼ cup baking soda
- 5 to 10 drops essential oil such as tea tree oil, jasmine oil, sandalwood oil, or any other oil that you find pleasing

Combine all ingredients well (either by hand or using a handheld emulsion mixer).

Store in an airtight container in your medicine cabinet or on your vanity, and apply under your arms using a small amount on the tips of your fingers. Feel free to make a half batch of this if you'd like to try it first.

Yields 1 cup.

Luxurious Coconut Oil Soap

This is just a basic soap recipe to get you started. It only makes a small batch so that if you make an error, you're not going to waste a large amount of product or money. Feel free to add in your choice of essential oils before pouring into molds if you'd like. You're going to be working with lye, which can be found next to drain cleaners at your local supermarket, so be careful because it's caustic. It's only used to cause the chemical reaction that makes soap, so the end product is perfectly safe.

- 2½ ounces lye
- 1 cup distilled water
- 5 ounces vegetable shortening
- 6 ounces virgin olive oil
- 6 ounces coconut oil, refined or virgin, depending on whether you want the smell
- ½ teaspoon essential oils of your choice

Make sure you're wearing safety glasses and gloves because this first step is a bit of a chemistry experiment. Combine the lye and water in a glass jar and stir until dissolved. The chemical reaction will heat the mixture up quickly, so be prepared. When it's dissolved, place the jar in a sink of ice water to cool it down to exactly 95 degrees F.

Melt the shortening in a medium-size stainless steel pot over medium heat. The pot must be stainless steel because the lye will interact with aluminum or other surfaces. Once the shortening is melted, add the olive oil and coconut oil, and heat until the oils reach exactly 95 degrees F.

Double-checking to be sure that both ingredients are at 95 degrees F, slowly pour the lye mixture into the oil, stirring constantly until it begins to "trace." This means that when you drag a spoon through it, a slight impression is left behind.

Add essential oils and mix thoroughly. You may also add a drop or two of food coloring at this point if you'd like.

Pour into molds and allow to cool for 24 hours. Then release and cut into bars. It will take up to a month for the bars to completely harden.

Yields about 6 bars of soap.

Coconut Oil Toothpaste

Coconut oil is thought to help prevent plaque buildup and tooth decay because of the antimicrobials in it, and baking soda has been used for eons as a cleansing agent, though the flavor isn't that great. That's why we're adding the mint!

- 2 teaspoons virgin coconut oil
- 3 drops peppermint oil
- 1 tablespoon baking soda

Add all three ingredients together and use just like you'd use regular toothpaste.

Yields almost 2 tablespoons.

Coconut Oil for Weight Loss

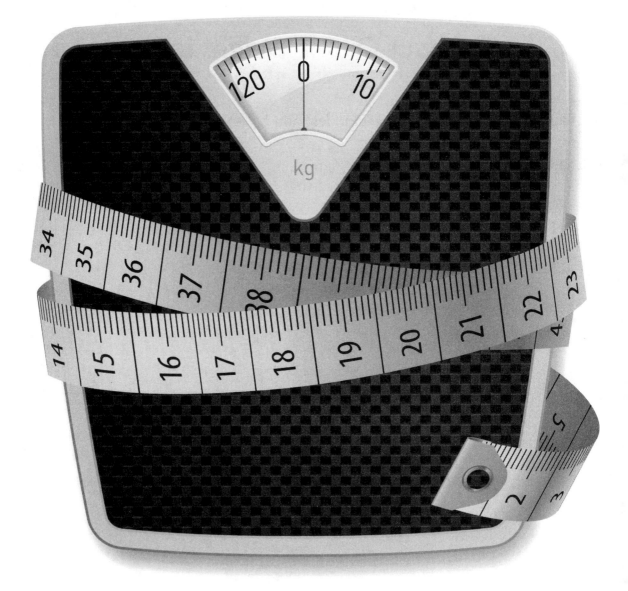

HOW COCONUT OIL CAN HELP YOU LOSE WEIGHT

Remember back in Chapter 3 when we were talking about the difference between medium-chain triglycerides (MCTs) and long-chain triglycerides (LCTs)? We discussed how MCTs are easily digested and used primarily as an energy source, whereas LCTs are more difficult to digest and are often stored as fat. This distinction makes all the difference in the world when it comes to finding ways to reach and maintain a healthy weight.

Good Fat Versus Bad Fat

Before we really get into the weight-loss benefits, we need to get past the negative press about saturated fats. The complaint about saturated fats versus unsaturated fats is that saturated fats raise your low-density lipoprotein (LDL), or "bad" cholesterol levels, thus leading to plaque buildup and other factors that cause heart disease. Since people who are overweight are already at a higher risk of heart disease, it's understandable that reducing saturated fats as part of a healthy weight-loss plan is the norm.

What makes coconut oil different? Although it's true that the MCTs in coconut oil are saturated fat, all saturated fats are not made the same. Unlike other saturated fats such as trans fats, medium-chain fatty acids raise both LDL cholesterol *and* high-density lipoprotein (HDL), or "good" cholesterol levels. Since HDL is responsible for carrying bad cholesterol out of the body, the saturated fats in coconut oil have little to no net effect on LDL cholesterol levels.

Now that the medical complaint for using coconut oil is out of the way, let's move on to the ways that coconut oil can help you lose weight and keep it off.

Improved Thyroid Function

Coconut oil's effect on thyroid function is actually more about what it doesn't do as opposed to what it does do. Hydrogenated oils, such as refined vegetable oils, can block protein absorption in the stomach, which, in turn, leads to hormonal changes that can affect thyroid function. In addition, these refined oils can also cause a decrease in thyroid function because they block hormone secretion, which can really sabotage your weight-loss efforts as well as your health. Signs of a poorly functioning thyroid include:

- Chronic fatigue
- Cold hands and feet
- Constipation
- Difficulty gaining or losing weight
- Difficulty sleeping
- Thinning hair
- Sleep disruptions, such as insomnia
- Depression
- Anxiety

MCTs such as the ones found in coconut oil don't do any of these bad things. Your thyroid is free to function as it was made to do.

Increased Metabolism

Without a doubt, coconut oil increases your metabolism, at least temporarily. The reason, again, is the way that your body rapidly breaks down and uses MCTs. Everything that your body does requires calories, or energy. Digesting the food that you eat typically takes about 10 percent of the calories that you ingest just to break them down and convert them to energy.

MCTs are pretty much shuttled straight to your liver because they're broken down very easily, so they don't consume the energy that the harder-to-digest LCTs do. Your body now has extra energy that it can use for, well, energy. It's estimated that MCTs take about one-third fewer calories to digest than other fats, thus increasing your metabolism.

In a recent research study of people who followed similar diets, the group that used coconut oil lost an average of seven pounds in a three-month period, while those who used other oils lost an average of only three pounds. The researchers suggested that the metabolic boost was perhaps caused by easy digestion of the coconut oil.

Another study evaluated the effect of MCTs on metabolism by measuring participants' metabolisms before and after consuming coconut oil. The average increase in metabolism for the group was 48 percent, but in obese participants, metabolism increased as much as 65 percent, and the fat-burning effect lasted as long as twenty-four hours.

Increased Energy Without Insulin Spikes

One of the biggest barriers to following a healthy diet is avoiding cravings and not feeling hungry all the time. Insulin spikes and food cravings are a direct result of how your body processes carbohydrates. They're easily broken down into glucose, which is your body's primary preferred source of energy. However, when you eat carbohydrates, either simple or complex, your blood is flooded with glucose, which causes your body to release insulin to absorb it.

Thus, your body gets a big burst of glucose . . . then an insulin spike to absorb it . . . then a huge energy crash because there's no longer any sugar in your bloodstream. Now you're going to crave more sugar for energy. MCTs like those found specifically in coconut oil are easily converted into quick energy but don't require the release of insulin to be used. Therefore, you're not going to get the peaks and crashes in your energy levels. Instead, you'll have a steady flow of energy to keep you going without getting cravings and without risking developing insulin resistance that can lead to type 2 diabetes.

Coconut Oil and Weight Loss

Regardless of what diet you're following, there is no instant magic pill, oil, or powder. When it comes right down to it, losing weight is a numbers game; if you burn more calories than you take in, you're going to lose weight. That being said, if you don't eat properly, you're not going to be able to successfully lose weight and stay healthy for the long-term. Incorporating coconut oil into your diet as a replacement for unhealthy saturated fats is a great way to get your figure ready for summer!

Speaking of healthy eating habits, it's easier to lose weight if you have a well-defined, healthy, weight-loss plan. We're going to help you out with that in the next chapter.

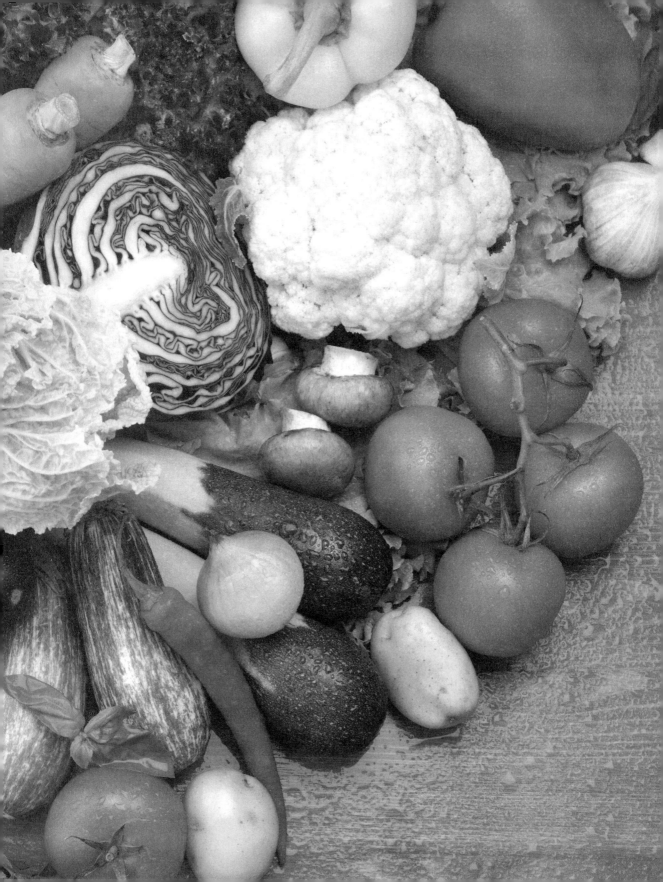

9

THE COCONUT OIL DIET PLAN

Losing weight isn't easy, as evidenced by the more than one-third of American adults who are struggling with obesity. According to the Centers for Disease Control and Prevention, obesity-related medical costs run about $147 billion per year and keep rising. Unfortunately, obesity doesn't just affect people physically; it's a social disease that affects everything from a person's interactions with others to employment opportunities.

Perhaps the saddest part is that obesity in our country is directly related to the Western lifestyle. As a matter of fact, diseases such as obesity, heart disease, diabetes, and stroke are often referred to as Western diseases or diseases of affluence. They're rarely seen in people who follow traditional Eastern or Mediterranean diets rich in omega-3s, vegetables, fruits, fish, lean meats, and medium-chain triglycerides (MCTs). These diets are also naturally low in processed and refined foods and bad fats.

Coconut Tip

Modern athletes often use MCTs instead of simple carbohydrates as a form of instant energy because they provide more sustained energy without the crash.

Throughout this chapter, we're going to map out a plan to help you shed those unhealthy, unsightly pounds for good without starving or running a marathon. No matter how much weight you need to lose, you're going to have a solid plan to meet your goals by the time we're done. There are three distinct areas that you're going to be addressing on your journey:

- Eliminating (or drastically reducing) "bad" foods that are making you obese
- Introducing delicious, good-for-you foods that promote health
- Increasing your activity levels

Remember that the road to good health is a marathon, not a sprint. You're going to fall down sometimes and you're going to falter. Just remember that you're not depriving yourself of ice cream; you're rewarding yourself with an attractive body that can do the things that you want to do. Here are a few tips to help you get through:

Be strict but gentle. If you occasionally falter, just move ahead. Don't beat yourself up . . . as long as you don't make a habit of cheating.

- Replace boredom or habitual eating with other behaviors that aren't compatible with eating, such as going for a walk, talking to a friend on the phone, or cleaning house.
- Eat small meals every couple of hours that have proteins and MCTs so that your blood-sugar levels stay stable.
- Don't focus on weight loss while you're breaking your sugar addiction and retraining yourself to eat healthily. It'll happen.

Let's start at the beginning and review some of the foods that you're going to want to ditch in order to begin your journey to a healthier, leaner you.

Step 1: Eliminate the Junk

Without a doubt, the hardest part of dieting is giving up the foods you love. We're going to let you in on a little secret, though: Once you break your sugar addiction and get the hang of eating right, you're going to develop a whole new list of favorites. The problem is that many of the foods that you *think* are good for you actually aren't.

Everybody knows that potato chips and snack cakes make you obese, but what about the canola oil or the "light" margarine that's supposedly the healthier alternative to butter? And what about the "light" microwave popcorn, fast-food "healthy" salads, sugar-free coffee creamer, or veggie chips? They all contain hydrogenated trans fats that not only make you obese but can quite literally kill you.

Where to Start

They say that every journey begins with a single step, and in this case, that step is ridding your home and your body of all of the fattening foods that will tempt you to cheat. Just remember, when you cheat, the only person that you're cheating is you! Here are a few tips to get you started:

- Look at your food labels and discard anything with hydrogenated fats or trans fats. Better yet, skip anything with a label and eat fresh fruits, veggies, dairy, and meats prepared with coconut oil.
- "Diet" drinks are just as bad for you as their sugar-laden cousins. They also trick your brain into thinking that you're getting sugar and can thus increase your sugar cravings. Drink water, coffee, or unsweetened tea. An occasional small glass of juice is OK, but limit it because you're basically drinking a glass of sugar without the beneficial fiber found in the fruit.
- Skip fried foods when you eat out. Chances are good that they're fried in hydrogenated oil.
- If you order a salad when eating out, use lemon juice to dress it instead of dressings. They're likely made with hydrogenated vegetable oils.
- Empty your pantry of junk food and refined foods such as white pastas, sugar, chips, cakes, and cookies. Do the same thing with your fridge.

Now that you know what you need to get rid of, let's move on and talk about what you need to start doing in order to successfully lose weight and get healthy.

Step 2: Introduce Delicious, Good-for-You Foods

This is the easy part because the only foods that you should avoid are the ones that are refined, processed, and full of trans fats and sugars. For the most part, when you go to the grocery store, you're going to be shopping the perimeter of the store. Rarely will you need to venture down an aisle, and when you do, get in and get out fast. Here's a list of good things to get you started:

- Brightly colored veggies
- Fruits, especially citrus fruits, apples, and berries
- Coconut oil, both virgin and naturally refined
- Lean meats
- Eggs
- Low-fat dairy products, if you're so inclined

Shop for a variety of foods so that you don't get bored. Also, shoot for a variety of colors because different colored fruits and veggies offer a variety of vitamins and nutrients. Don't buy protein bars or other so-called health foods. Just buy natural, unprocessed foods that are as close to their natural state as possible. This does, of course, include plenty of both virgin and naturally refined coconut oils to replace those other fats that are making you pudgy.

OK, now that you have a rough guideline of what you're going to be eating, let's talk for a minute about exercise. Don't moan—you're going to be surprised by some of the fun things that you can do to increase your activity levels.

Step 3: Increase Activity Levels

Like we've already discussed, losing weight is a numbers game; if you burn more calories than you eat, you're going to lose weight. Also, if you're exercising, you're not eating! How much you'll be able to exercise depends on your physical abilities. If you have a large amount of weight to lose and simply cannot get out and play a crazy game of beach volleyball, at least go for a walk around your neighborhood. Here are a few quick ways to easily increase your activity levels and thus burn more calories:

- Park in the farthest parking spot away from the store and walk.
- Take the stairs instead of the elevator.
- Take a walk at lunch instead of taking the entire time to eat. Do the same with your morning and afternoon breaks.
- Go window shopping at the mall. If you have to buy something, park so that you're walking the length of the mall or supermarket to get to what you need.
- Organize a nightly neighborhood walk.
- Take your dog for an extra walk.
- Do squats or toe raises while standing in line instead of standing still.
- Schedule an exercise date such as a walk, hike, or bike ride instead of planning a dinner out.

Regardless of your fitness level, there are a million things you can do to increase your activity levels and thus burn more calories. The bottom line, however, is that if you're not eating the right foods, you can exercise all you want and still not get that beach body you're working so hard for. The next section features some delicious recipes that include coconut oil, which offers you those wonderful, fat-burning MCTs.

Now it's time for the recipes. Coconut oil's benefits can be enjoyed at any meal of the day from breakfast to after-dinner dessert, so get ready for some surprising, healthy, and tasty recipes!

SECTION FIVE

Coconut Oil Recipes

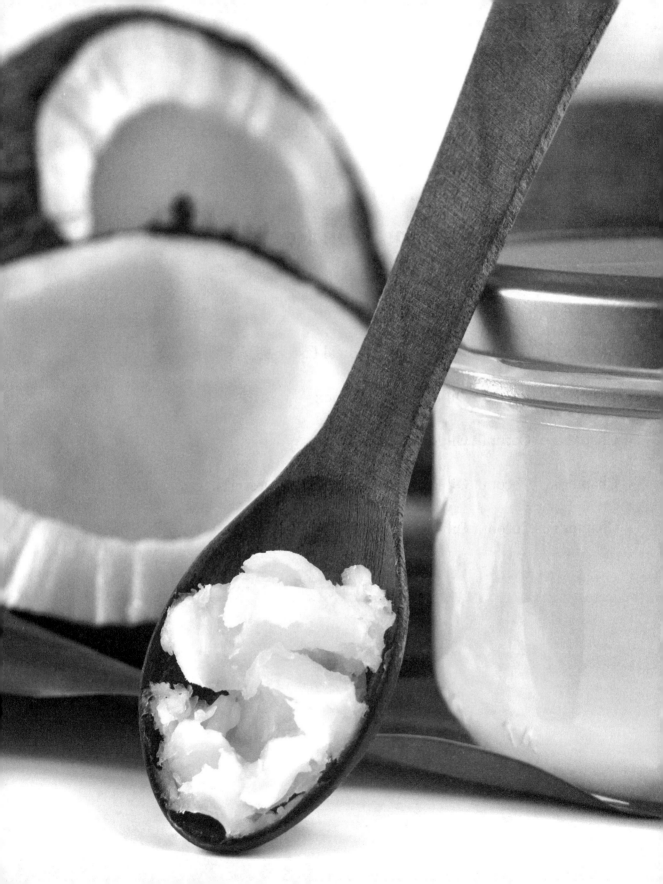

COOKING WITH COCONUT OIL

Since saturated fats have been ostracized by Western health care professionals for the past twenty years or so, chances are good that you've never even seen coconut oil, let alone cooked with it. Relax though; this is the easy part. After we touch on a few basic points, you'll be using it like a pro and wondering why you didn't make the switch ages ago. Why? Because coconut oil is not just healthy, it's delicious.

Coconut Oil Basics

There are a few things that you need to know before you get started, but for the most part, coconut oil is one of the easiest fats on the planet to work with because you can substitute it in equal parts for any other fat out there, regardless of whether it's liquid or solid.

Coconut Quick Fact

Because its melting temperature is about 76 degrees Fahrenheit, which is roughly room temperature, coconut oil fluctuates from liquid to solid easily and frequently. Unlike other oils, quality isn't affected when this happens and refrigeration isn't necessary. As a matter of fact, if you refrigerate coconut oil, it gets as hard as a rock!

To melt coconut oil, measure out the desired amount and heat it gently in the microwave, on the stove, or by setting the entire jar in warm water. Here are some tips to help you work with the unusual liquid and solid states of coconut oil:

- Have your other ingredients at room temperature if you're using coconut oil in liquid form.

- If you're heating your oil up to a liquid state, heat your other liquid ingredients with it so that they don't cool it back down enough to resolidify.

- If you want the liquid form, wait until you have your other ingredients mixed together and then quickly whisk in your melted coconut oil, along with any other liquid ingredients that you heated.

Virgin or Refined

Although many people will insist that virgin is the only healthy way to go, there are refining methods such as the ones discussed in Section 1 that don't negatively impact the oil. Just make sure that if you use a refined oil, it's refined without the use of chemicals.

The only real culinary difference between virgin and refined coconut oils is the flavor. Virgin coconut oil will have a rich, nutty, coconutty flavor that you'll need to keep in mind when you're putting together flavor profiles. Refined coconut oil has no coconut flavor; the only way you'll know that you're using refined coconut oil is that your food will often have a much more attractive, crispy sear. Also, coconut oil doesn't tend to weigh food down the way that butter or vegetable oil does.

We recommend keeping both virgin and refined coconut oil on hand.

Baking with Coconut Oil

You can substitute coconut oil for solid fats such as vegetable shortening or lard in recipes. Just use equal parts. It makes an amazingly light, crispy pie or pastry crust, and your biscuits will have a pleasant, nongreasy texture and a beautiful brown crown. You can also substitute coconut oil for liquid vegetable oil with no negative impact. Just follow the melting directions given earlier.

Frying with Coconut Oil

Keep flavor profiles in mind when you're choosing between virgin and refined coconut oil, but that's the only functionally significant difference between the two when it comes to cooking.

The smoke point of virgin coconut oil is 350 degrees Fahrenheit, the exact same temperature as butter. Comparatively, refined coconut oil has a smoke point of up to 450 degrees Fahrenheit, extra-virgin olive oil has a smoke point of about 320 degrees Fahrenheit, and most refined vegetable oils range from 220 to 430 degrees Fahrenheit. In other words, coconut oil is comparable to other oils regardless of whether it's refined or virgin.

We recommend choosing virgin or refined based upon whether or not you want to add sweet coconut notes to your dish. This may be great with something like tropical fish dishes but perhaps not so fabulous if you're making Grandma's Chicken Parmesan.

Using Coconut Oil Raw

Many people thoroughly enjoy using coconut oil as a butter replacement, whether as a spread for toast or as part of a recipe for dips, spreads, or even cake icing. It's also great as the oil base for salad dressings such as vinaigrettes. Its uses are limited only by your imagination!

You should now officially have a handle on how to cook with coconut oil, so let's move on to the recipes.

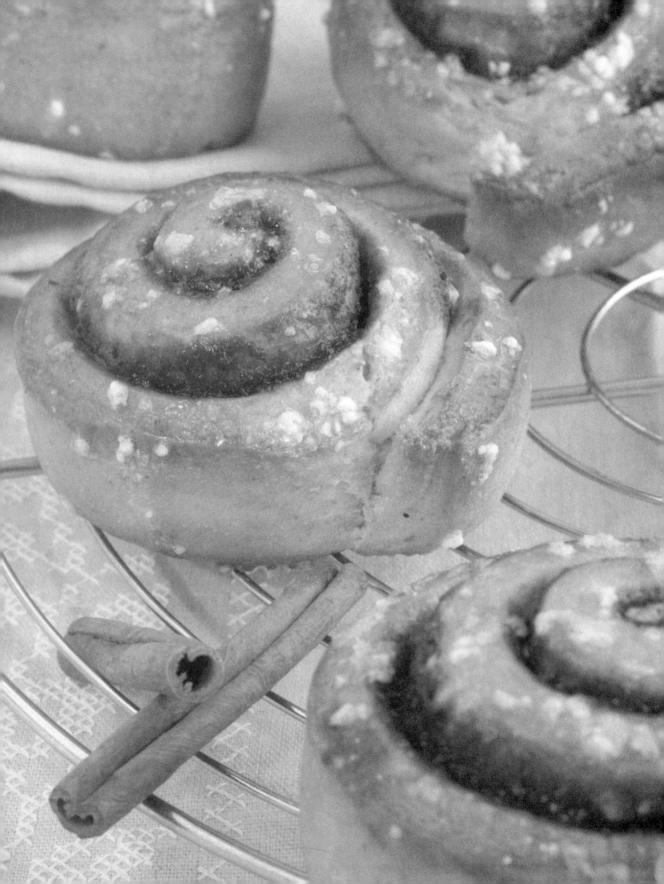

COCONUT OIL RECIPES FOR BREAKFAST

Fluffy Coconut Pancakes

You have a couple of options here—if you'd like to make traditional pancakes that are mouthwateringly delicious, use refined coconut oil. If you'd like to lend an exotic flair to them, use virgin coconut oil. Whatever you choose, these pancakes are going to be a hit!

- 2 cups all-purpose flour
- 1½ tablespoons granulated sugar
- 2 teaspoons baking powder
- 1 teaspoon salt
- 2 eggs, beaten
- 1½ cups whole or 2% milk, at room temperature
- ¼ cup + 2 teaspoons virgin or refined coconut oil, melted and divided

In a medium mixing bowl, combine your dry ingredients. Then add the eggs, milk, and ¼ cup of coconut oil. Stir only enough to combine the ingredients or else your pancakes will be tough. There will still be lumps in the batter.

Preheat a medium skillet or griddle, and grease with part of the remaining coconut oil. Add pancake batter ¼ cup at a time. Fry on one side until bubbles form across the top of the pancake and the edges begin to look dry. Flip and fry for an additional minute or until brown. Remove and keep warm in a heated oven until you're finished cooking.

Yields about 8 (6-inch) pancakes.

Mediterranean Omelet

Light and fluffy, this omelet is a great way to get a healthy start to your day. If you'd like to make it even healthier, just use the egg whites.

- 1 teaspoon refined coconut oil
- 3 eggs, whipped
- 2 tablespoons diced tomatoes
- 1 tablespoon chopped red onion
- ¼ cup sliced mushrooms
- 10 spinach leaves
- 2 tablespoons crumbled feta cheese

Preheat a medium skillet over medium heat and grease with the coconut oil. Once the skillet is hot, pour in the eggs, and then add the vegetables.

When the top of the eggs begin to look dry, add the feta cheese and fold the omelet in half. Remove from the pan and enjoy!

Yields 1 omelet.

Southern Style Country Biscuits

If you like flaky, home-style biscuits, then you're going to love what coconut oil does to this recipe. For that matter, if you have a favorite biscuit recipe of your own, try substituting coconut oil for the fat and see what a difference it makes. Hint: They'll be flakier and have a beautiful golden crust and sweet flavor without being greasy. You'll never switch back! The key to fluffy biscuits is in the mixing. Don't stir the dough any more than you absolutely have to.

- ⅔ cup + 1 tablespoon refined coconut oil, divided
- 4 cups all-purpose flour
- 2 tablespoons baking powder
- 1 teaspoon salt
- 1 tablespoon granulated sugar
- 1½ cups milk
- 2 eggs, beaten

Preheat oven to 400 degrees F, and grease a cookie sheet with 1 teaspoon of the coconut oil.

In a medium mixing bowl, combine all of the dry ingredients and add ⅔ cup of coconut oil. Cut the mixture with a pastry cutter until you have pea-sized lumps evenly distributed.

Whisk the milk into the eggs, and then add to the dry mixture. Stir until moistened, and then turn out onto a floured surface.

Knead as little as possible—no more than 20 times. Roll out so that the dough is about 1 inch thick, and cut using a biscuit cutter or a floured drinking cup.

Place the cut dough on the cookie sheet with the sides touching, and brush the tops with the remaining coconut oil. Bake for 10 to 15 minutes or until tops are golden brown.

Yields about 18 biscuits.

Island Style Banana Nut Muffins

Typical muffins are laden with artery-clogging butter, but these moist, light muffins are great for an occasional breakfast treat because they're made with healthy coconut oil. Make sure your bananas are as ripe as possible, as that's when they're most flavorful. As a matter of fact, making these muffins is a great way to avoid wasting those overripe bananas that nobody will eat.

- 4 ripe bananas
- 1 cup granulated sugar
- 2 eggs
- ¾ cup virgin coconut oil

- 2 cups all-purpose flour
- 2 teaspoons baking soda
- ¾ teaspoon salt
- ½ cup walnuts

Preheat oven to 350 degrees F. Line 12 muffin cups with cupcake papers and set aside.

In a medium bowl, mash your bananas until they're smooth. Add the sugar and eggs, and beat for 2 to 3 minutes or until the sugar is dissolved. Add the coconut oil and continue to mix for another minute.

In a separate medium bowl, combine the flour, baking soda, and salt. Then add to the banana mixture and mix for 1 more minute. Stir in the nuts and spoon the batter into the cupcake papers until they're about two-thirds full.

Bake for 20 minutes or until a toothpick inserted in the middle comes out clean.

Yields about 12 muffins.

Ooey Gooey Cinnamon Rolls

Again, you have the option of choosing whether or not you'd like to maintain a traditional flavor by using refined coconut oil or if you'd like to be a bit exotic and use the virgin oil to lend the coconut flavor. Either way, you're going to love them!

- ¼ cup warm water
- 1 packet instant yeast
- ¾ cup whole or 2% milk
- 1 cup virgin or refined coconut oil, divided
- 3½ cups all-purpose flour, divided
- 1½ tablespoons cinnamon, divided
- ¼ cup granulated sugar
- ½ teaspoon salt
- 1 egg
- 1 cup packed dark brown sugar
- ½ cup chopped pecans

Put the warm water in a small bowl and add the yeast.

In a small saucepan, heat milk and ⅓ cup of coconut oil until it starts to simmer. Stir to mix and remove from heat.

In a large mixing bowl, combine half of the flour, ½ tablespoon cinnamon, and all of the granulated sugar and salt. Mix well, and add the water and yeast as well as the milk mixture and the egg. Mix in the remaining flour ¼ cup at a time until the dough loses its stickiness.

When the dough is blended, turn it out onto a lightly floured surface. Knead until the dough is smooth and elastic, about 5 to 6 minutes.

Place the dough in a medium bowl and cover with a warm, damp towel for about 15 minutes.

While the dough is resting, combine the remaining cinnamon, coconut oil, and brown sugar in a bowl.

Roll the dough out into a rectangle until it's about ½ inch thick. Spread the brown sugar mixture onto the dough and sprinkle with the pecans. If you've opted for virgin coconut oil, some coconut flakes might be nice, too.

Starting at a wide side, begin rolling the dough into a log. Slice the log in 1-inch-thick pieces, and place them on a cookie sheet greased with coconut oil so that the sides touch. Cover and place in a warm place until they rise to twice their original size.

Bake for 20 minutes or until lightly browned. Cool and enjoy!

Yields 1 dozen rolls.

Southwest Breakfast Wrap

These wraps are a great on-the-go breakfast and can even be made ahead of time and frozen. Whether you're late for work or heading out on a weekend hike, the protein and medium-chain triglycerides (MCTs) in this wrap will get you through.

- 6 eggs
- 3 tablespoons chopped ham
- 1 green pepper, chopped
- 2 tablespoons chopped red onion

- 3 (8-inch) whole-wheat tortillas
- 1 tablespoon refined coconut oil
- ¼ cup pepper jack cheese

Preheat oven to 350 degrees F. Whisk all ingredients, except the wraps, coconut oil, and cheese, together in a medium bowl.

Put the tortillas in the oven for about 5 minutes and warm them up while you're cooking the eggs. Remove when they're warm.

Heat a medium frying pan greased with coconut oil over medium heat, and add the egg mixture when the skillet is hot. Stir slowly until eggs are thoroughly cooked. Place wraps on a clean cutting board side by side. Divide the egg mixture between them and top with cheese.

Fold 1 side of the tortilla over the egg mixture. Fold ends in, and then continue to roll.

Yields 3 wraps.

Southern Breakfast Hash

This old-fashioned, stick-to-your-ribs breakfast is great for weekends or for when you have company and want to cook a large amount of food with little fuss. It's everything that you need, all in one skillet. The proteins and healthy fat will have you running all morning.

- 2 tablespoons refined coconut oil
- 6 potatoes, peeled and shredded
- ½ teaspoon salt
- ½ teaspoon black pepper
- 1½ cups cubed breakfast ham
- ½ red onion, sliced
- 1 cup chopped mushrooms
- ½ cup shredded cheese, or more if you prefer
- 6 eggs

Heat a large skillet over medium heat and add coconut oil. When the oil is hot, add the potatoes, salt, and pepper and let cook until potatoes start to brown.

Add the ham, onions, and mushrooms and continue to fry, stirring as needed until the potatoes are brown and the veggies are tender. Top with cheese.

In a separate skillet, soft fry the eggs and place on top of the potato mixture.

Yields 6 servings.

Orange Coconut French Toast

It's time to see what this coconut oil can really do. Let's mix up some decadent French toast using more of the healthy coastal coconut than just the oil. We can't really call this dish healthy, but by replacing the butter with the coconut oil, it's certainly better for you than the traditional version.

- 2 eggs
- ½ cup unsweetened coconut milk
- ¼ cup orange juice
- 1 tablespoon orange zest
- ½ teaspoon cinnamon
- ¼ teaspoon almond extract
- 1 pinch sea salt

- 1 tablespoon + 1 teaspoon virgin coconut oil, divided
- 4 slices of brioche bread
- 2 teaspoons unsweetened coconut flakes
- 4 slices of orange
- Syrup or fruit topping

In a medium bowl, combine the eggs, coconut milk, orange juice, orange zest, cinnamon, almond extract, and salt. Whisk together until well mixed.

Heat a large skillet over medium heat, and melt 1 tablespoon coconut oil in it. Dip each piece of bread in the egg mixture, soaking for about 20 seconds. Remove and let drain for a couple of seconds, and then place in the hot skillet. Cook each slice for about 3 minutes on each side, until it's brown.

Remove from heat and place two slices on each plate. Brush with remaining teaspoon of coconut oil. Garnish with coconut flakes and orange slices. Top with your favorite syrup or fruit topping.

Yields 2 servings.

Coconut-Banana Waffles

With this variation on the use of traditional flours, you'll get the full coconut experience! Mashed bananas make these waffles perfectly moist and sweet, and walnuts add some crunch. Think banana bread in a waffle iron. These freeze well, so make extra to reheat on other busy mornings.

- 1 cup coconut flour
- 1/2 cup tapioca flour
- 1 teaspoon baking soda
- 1/4 teaspoon salt
- 1/2 cup chopped walnuts
- 4 large eggs, beaten
- 1/2 cup mashed ripe banana
- 1/4 cup plain coconut milk
- 2 tablespoons virgin coconut oil, melted
- 1 teaspoon vanilla extract

In a large mixing bowl, stir together the coconut and tapioca flours, baking soda, salt, and walnuts until well blended.

In a separate bowl, mix together the eggs, mashed banana, coconut milk, coconut oil, and vanilla, then stir into the dry ingredients. Using a hand mixer, mix on low speed until well blended. Set aside for 10 minutes while heating a waffle iron.

Ladle batter into the waffle iron and cook according to manufacturer's instructions. As each waffle is finished, transfer it to a covered dish to keep warm.

To serve, top the warm waffles with maple syrup or fruit.

Yields 4 waffles.

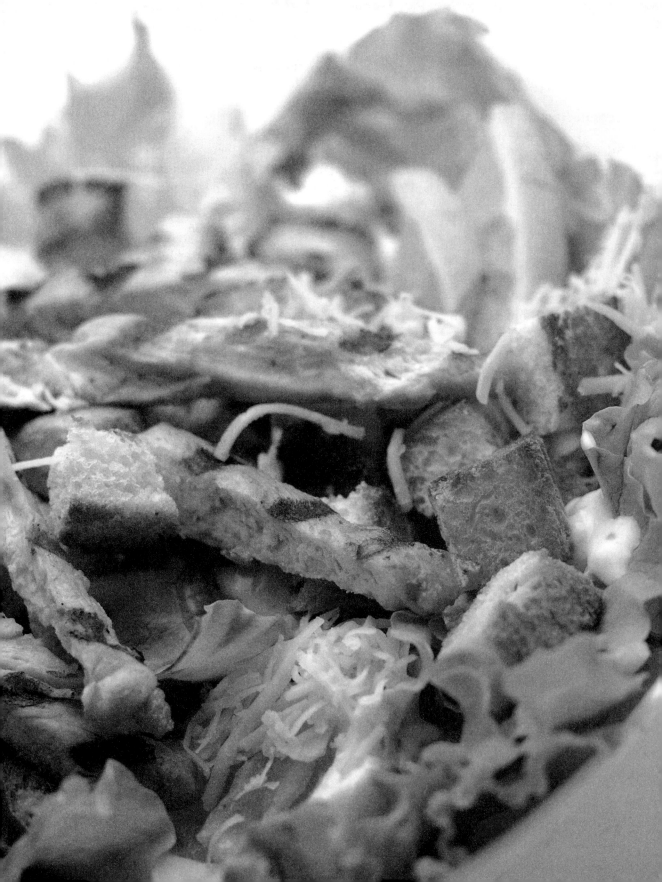

COCONUT OIL RECIPES FOR LUNCH

Buffalo Bison Burger

This juicy, delicious burger is made even better by the addition of coconut oil, both in the burger and the sauce. Because bison tends to be a bit too lean to make a juicy burger, it's often mixed with other fattier meats. In this case, the coconut oil does the trick so you can eat the leaner meat without the added "bad" saturated fat.

- 1 pound ground bison meat
- 3 tablespoons virgin coconut oil, divided
- 1 teaspoon sea salt
- 1 teaspoon black pepper
- 4 tablespoons hot sauce
- 1 teaspoon vinegar
- 1 pinch garlic powder
- Dash of Worcestershire sauce
- 4 hamburger buns
- 2 tablespoons blue cheese crumbles

Preheat grill to medium heat. Place the bison meat in a medium bowl, and add 2 tablespoons of the coconut oil and the salt and pepper. Mix thoroughly. Separate into 4 patties and place on the grill.

While the meat is cooking, mix the remaining coconut oil in a small saucepan with the hot sauce, vinegar, Worcestershire sauce, and garlic powder. Whisk to blend, and heat just until hot.

When the burgers are done, drizzle the sauce over, place them on the buns, and top with blue cheese crumbles. Garnish as you'd like.

Yields 4 burgers.

Coconut Mango Salad with Chicken

This crispy green salad is packed full of nutrients and is deliciously light, as well. Don't worry though—the combination of chicken, nuts, and coconut oil will ensure that it holds you over until your next meal.

Chicken

- 1 teaspoon virgin coconut oil
- 1 boneless, skinless chicken breast
- 1 pinch salt
- 1 pinch black pepper

Salad

- 1 cup mixed baby greens
- 1 cup baby spinach
- 1 tablespoon chopped walnuts

- 1 tablespoon chopped mango
- 1 tablespoon dried cranberries
- 1 tablespoon chopped red onion
- 1 tablespoon feta cheese

Dressing

- 1 tablespoon coconut oil
- 1 tablespoon balsamic vinegar
- 1 teaspoon orange juice

Heat a small skillet over medium heat and add 1 teaspoon of coconut oil. When the skillet is hot, add the chicken breast and sprinkle with the salt and pepper. Cook 4 minutes on each side or until the meat is no longer pink. Remove from heat and set aside.

Toss the salad ingredients in a bowl together and place on a large plate.

For the dressing, heat the coconut oil, balsamic vinegar, and orange juice together in a small saucepan until the coconut oil melts.

Place the chicken breast on top of the salad and drizzle with the dressing.

Yields 1 serving.

Coconut Caesar Dressing

This recipe adds a bit of the exotic to a classic dressing. If you'd rather have a more traditional flavor, feel free to use refined coconut oil instead of virgin.

- 3 anchovy filets, rinsed
- 1 egg
- 1 egg white
- 2 cloves of garlic, minced
- 2 tablespoons lemon juice
- 1 pinch salt
- 1 pinch black pepper
- ¼ teaspoon Worcestershire sauce
- ¼ cup virgin or refined coconut oil, melted

Make a paste from the anchovies by smashing them with the back of a spoon.

Place the paste in a medium bowl, and mix in the egg, egg white, minced garlic, lemon juice, salt, pepper, and Worcestershire sauce. Continue to mix briskly and slowly add in the melted coconut oil. Continue to mix until the mixture is completely emulsified. Use as a traditional Caesar dressing, or baste white-fleshed fish or chicken with it.

Yields ⅔ cup.

Coconut Granola Bars

These are great for a meal on the run or for a snack to hold you over. They're rich in both healthy fats and fiber, so they'll provide sustained energy to get you through a hectic workday or an active Saturday of hiking.

- 2 cups rolled oats
- ½ cup toasted mixed nuts, chopped
- ¼ cup virgin coconut oil, melted
- ⅓ cup local organic honey
- ½ cup unsweetened coconut flakes
- ½ cup dried dates, chopped
- ½ teaspoon cinnamon
- ¼ teaspoon sea salt
- ½ cup dried pineapple

Preheat oven to 350 degrees F, and line a cookie sheet with parchment paper. Put the oats and the nuts into a mixing bowl and drizzle the coconut oil over them. Toss until coated and spread on the cookie sheet. Bake for 10 minutes, stir, and then bake for another 10 minutes.

While they're toasting, put the honey in a small saucepan and bring to a boil over medium heat. Reduce heat and simmer for 5 more minutes. Remove from heat.

Place the oat and nut mixture along with the other dry ingredients in a large mixing bowl, and mix with your hands until well combined. Drizzle the honey over the nuts and grains, and stir gently to coat. Press onto a cookie sheet greased with coconut oil, and place in the oven. Bake for 25 to 30 minutes or until lightly browned.

Spread the mayo on the roll, and cut into 2 x 4–inch bars. Store in an airtight container for up to 1 week.

Yields 10 bars.

Ham Sammy with Tropical Chipotle Mayo

This is truly a taste of the islands. Sweet ham grilled in pineapple juice and coconut oil with a sweet coconut oil chipotle mayo will take you straight from your office to an instant vacation. You'll practically feel sand between your toes.

- 2 teaspoons virgin coconut oil, melted
- ¼ pound thick-sliced breakfast ham
- 2 pineapple rings
- 1 ciabatta roll, sliced lengthwise
- 4 slices Roma tomato
- 15 spinach leaves
- 4 red onion rings
- 1 tablespoon Tropical Chipotle Mayo, recipe follows

Preheat a skillet or grill to medium heat. Brush the ham, pineapple, and roll with coconut oil and grill just enough to leave sear marks. Remove from grill.

Spread the mayo on the roll, and then add the ham, pineapple, tomato, spinach, and onion.

Yields 1 sandwich.

Tropical Chipotle Mayo

This mayo lacks the saturated fat of typical mayonnaise and has a nice kick that's sweetened up by the coconut oil. Use the virgin oil for this recipe—it truly does make the difference between good and great. Use it like a standard mayo or as a marinade for chicken or shrimp. It's even good as a dip for fried pickles.

- 1 teaspoon apple cider vinegar
- 2 teaspoons lemon juice
- 1 egg yolk
- ½ teaspoon Worcestershire sauce
- ½ teaspoon salt
- ½ tablespoon dry mustard
- ½ tablespoon cayenne pepper
- 1 cup virgin coconut oil, melted

In a small bowl, combine vinegar and lemon juice, and set aside. In a medium glass bowl, whisk together the egg yolk, Worcestershire sauce, and the dry ingredients. When they're combined, briskly whisk in half of the vinegar and lemon juice combination. When that's combined, start adding the coconut oil just a little bit at a time while continuously whisking vigorously.

When the mixture starts to look a little lighter and gets a little thicker, you can slow the whisking down a little because your mayo is emulsified. Add the rest of the lemon juice combination, and then continue to slowly add the oil until you're finished.

Allow to rest at room temperature for an hour or so and then refrigerate.

Yields about 1 cup.

Grilled Coconut Shrimp

This is quick and easy to make, and it's healthy, too. These shrimp are great to eat alone or to toss on top of a salad. Shrimp are also high in omega-3 fatty acids, so you're getting a real boost when you combine them with the power of coconut oil.

- 1 tablespoon virgin coconut oil
- 6 large shrimp, peeled and deveined
- 2 pinches paprika

Heat the coconut oil in a medium sauté pan at medium heat. When it's hot, add the shrimp to the oil and cook for about 1 minute on each side or until they curl. Remove from heat and sprinkle with the paprika. Serve as you'd like.

Yields 1 serving.

Coconut Grouper

This is great just by itself or on a sandwich, so take your pick! Grouper is a nice, light fish that lacks the "fishy" taste that turns many people away from fish. The coconut oil gives it a nice flavor as well as a golden crust. You can use refined coconut oil if you'd rather, but the virgin oil lends it a nice sweetness.

- ¼ cup coconut flour
- ¼ teaspoon salt
- ¼ teaspoon black pepper
- ¼ teaspoon paprika
- 1 tablespoon virgin or refined coconut oil
- 2 grouper filets
- 2 lemon wedges

Combine flour, salt, pepper, and paprika in a shallow bowl or on a plate. Heat coconut oil in a medium skillet over medium-high heat. Dredge grouper fillets in the flour mixture, and drop gently into the hot oil. Fry for about 2 minutes on each side depending upon the thickness of the fillets. The fish will flake when it's done.

Serve with a side or as a sandwich, and garnish with lemon wedges. The Tropical Chipotle Mayo presented earlier goes wonderfully with this dish.

Yields 2 servings.

Grilled Fruit and Veggie Medley

This is a great side dish or is delicious and nutritious as a stand-alone vegetarian dish. Brushed with seasoned coconut oil and grilled lightly, you may just have a new favorite dish. Feel free to substitute all of your favorite fruits and veggies if these don't work for you.

- 3 tablespoons virgin coconut oil
- 1 clove garlic, minced
- 12 cherry tomatoes
- 1 green pepper, chunked
- ½ cup brussels sprouts, halved
- ½ red onion, quartered
- ½ cup fresh pineapple, cut into 1-inch cubes
- ½ cup fresh mango, cut into 1-inch cubes
- ½ cup watermelon, cut into 1-inch cubes
- ⅛ teaspoon sea salt
- ½ teaspoon fresh chopped basil

In a large sauté pan, warm the coconut oil over medium-low heat. Add the garlic. Increase the heat to medium and add all of the veggies as well as the pineapple and mango. Toss to coat. Wait until the very end to add the watermelon, salt, and basil. Serve on a plate and enjoy.

Yields about 4 servings.

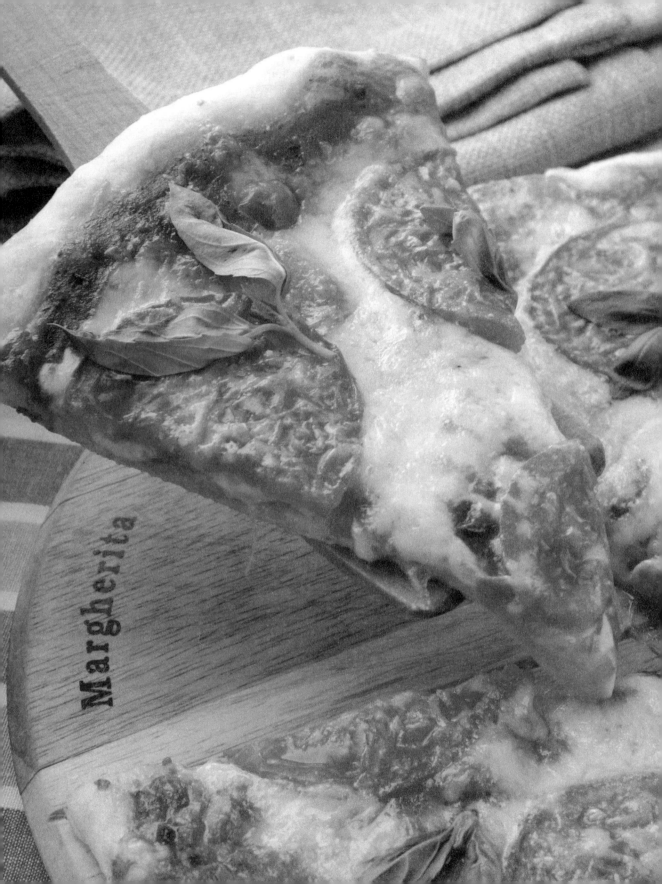

COCONUT OIL RECIPES FOR DINNER

Mango Salmon

Salmon is rich in omega-3s and is a staple in the Mediterranean diet because of its extensive health benefits. The salsa that we're going to make is packed with disease-fighting antioxidants, and the coconut oil lends a crispy texture and a sweet flavor to counteract some of the heat in the salsa.

- 2 tablespoons chopped tomato
- 2 tablespoons chopped mango
- 2 teaspoons chopped red onion
- 1 teaspoon chopped cilantro
- ½ teaspoon chopped jalapeño pepper
- 1 clove garlic, minced
- 1 tablespoon virgin coconut oil
- 2 (6-ounce) salmon filets
- ⅛ teaspoon sea salt

In a small bowl, add the tomato, mango, red onion, cilantro, jalapeño, and garlic, and stir well to combine. Set the salsa aside while you prepare the salmon.

Heat the coconut oil in a medium skillet over medium heat. When it's hot, add the salmon filets and sprinkle with the salt. Cook for about 3 minutes and turn. Cook for another 3 minutes and test for doneness, depending upon your preference.

Place the salmon on the plate and top with 2 tablespoons of the salsa.

Yields 2 servings.

Scallops and Angel Hair Pasta with a Coconut Cream Sauce

This dish may sound complicated, and all of your friends will think it is, but this simple sauce only tastes complex. Whip it up on a weeknight when you want something creamy and delicious but don't want to spend all night in the kitchen.

- 2 quarts salted water
- 1 cup unsweetened coconut milk
- 1 tablespoon ground thyme
- 1 tablespoon ground rosemary
- ½ teaspoon salt, divided

- ½ teaspoon black pepper
- ½ pound angel hair pasta
- 1 tablespoon virgin coconut oil
- 10 large sea scallops

Bring 2 quarts of salted water to a boil for the pasta. Put the coconut milk, thyme, rosemary, one half of the salt, and the pepper in a medium saucepan and bring to a boil. Lower heat to a simmer and reduce the sauce until it begins to thicken. Set aside.

Add pasta to the boiling water, and cook until tender.

Heat a medium skillet over medium heat and add the coconut oil. When it's hot, add the scallops and sprinkle with the remaining salt. Leave them alone until they get a nice, brown crust on the bottom, then turn. When the scallops brown, they're done. They will still be slightly translucent because they continue to cook when you remove them from the skillet.

Add the pasta to the scallop skillet and pour the sauce over the pasta. Toss to coat. Place onto two plates and top with 5 scallops each.

Yields 2 servings.

Coconut Pork Kabobs

Spicy pork kabobs are great for any summer barbecue or even for a simple Monday night dinner. The coconut oil and jerk seasoning lend the meat an exotic flair, while the oil helps sear the veggies to bring out their natural sweetness.

- 1 pound pork roast, cut into bite-sized cubes
- 1 tablespoon Caribbean jerk seasoning
- 2 tablespoons virgin coconut oil, divided
- 2 green peppers, cut into eighths
- ½ red onion, quartered
- 1 cup fresh or canned pineapple chunks

Rub the meat with the jerk seasoning and drizzle with 1 tablespoon of the coconut oil. Allow to sit for at least 15 minutes.

Preheat grill to medium-high heat. Alternately thread meat, veggies, and pineapple onto kabob skewers. Brush with the remaining coconut oil and place on the grill. Cook 1½ minutes on each side, turning one-quarter turn so that all four sides get a sear. Check meat for doneness and remove when veggies and meat are done.

Yields about 6 skewers.

Sizzling Beef Fajitas

You don't really want coconut flavoring in this Tex-Mex favorite, so use refined coconut oil for this recipe. The oil replaces less healthy vegetable oil, letting you enjoy this meal even more than you normally would.

- 8 small tortillas
- 2 tablespoons refined coconut oil
- 2 cloves garlic, minced
- 1 pound beef rib eye, cut into strips
- 1 teaspoon sea salt

- 1 teaspoon black pepper
- 3 green peppers, sliced
- 1 white onion, sliced
- Garnish of shredded lettuce, tomato, shredded cheese and sour cream

Heat up two fajita skillets in the oven at 400 degrees F while you're preparing the meal.

Wrap the tortillas in 4 separate aluminum foil packets, and place them in the oven when you add the veggies to the skillet in the steps that follow.

Heat 2 tablespoons of coconut oil in an extra large skillet and add the minced garlic. Add the steak strips, sprinkle with salt and pepper, and sear for 2 to 3 minutes or until meat is medium-rare. Add the peppers and onion, and toss together. Cook for another 2 to 3 minutes or until veggies are tender.

Divide the fajita mixture between the 4 plates. Serve family style along with the garnish and tortillas.

Yields 4 servings.

New York Strip with Coconut Horseradish Cream Sauce

The subtle taste of coconut in this dish tempers the flavor of the horseradish and pairs nicely with the blackened flavor of the steak.

- 2 medium New York strip steaks
- 2 tablespoons virgin coconut oil
- 2 tablespoons Cajun seasoning
- ½ cup unsweetened coconut milk
- 4 ounces goat cheese
- 2 tablespoons prepared horseradish

Coat the steaks with the coconut oil and Cajun seasoning, and let them sit while you make the sauce. Preheat the grill to medium-high.

Whisk the milk, cheese, and horseradish together to make a sauce.

Put the steaks on the grill and cook 4 to 6 minutes on each side for medium-rare.

Serve each steak with a dollop of sauce.

Yields 2 servings.

Coconut Beef Stir-Fry

Everybody loves a good stir-fry, but once you try it with coconut oil, you'll never go back to cooking with regular oil again. Keep your vegetables al dente because they'll lend a nice texture to your dish.

- 2 teaspoons garlic powder
- 3 tablespoons arrowroot powder, divided
- 3 tablespoons + ½ cup water, divided
- 1 pound boneless sirloin steak, cut into strips
- 2 tablespoons virgin coconut oil, divided

- 3 cups broccoli florets
- 1 cup snow peas
- ½ cup watercress
- ⅓ cup soy sauce
- 1½ tablespoons brown sugar
- ½ teaspoon ground ginger

In a medium bowl, make a paste from the garlic powder, 2 tablespoons of arrowroot powder, and 3 tablespoons of water. Put the beef in the bowl and toss to coat.

Heat 1 tablespoon of the coconut oil in a wok and add the steak strips. Stir-fry until nearly done and set aside. Add the other tablespoon of oil to the wok and toss in the veggies. Stir-fry until crisp-tender and add the beef to the veggies.

In a small bowl, mix the soy sauce, remaining arrowroot powder, brown sugar, ginger, and ½ cup water until dissolved. Pour over the steak and veggies. Toss to coat and heat for another minute.

Serve with rice or lo mein.

Yields 4 servings.

Grilled Coconut Blackened Chicken

The coconut oil lends a nice crispness to the outside of the breast while sealing the juices inside. This simple breast goes well over a nice dinner salad or as an entrée. Consider this a base grilled chicken recipe to build upon if you're in need of a quick chicken dish.

- 2 boneless, skinless chicken breasts
- 2 teaspoons blackening seasoning
- 3 teaspoons virgin coconut oil
- ⅛ teaspoon salt

Rub chicken breasts with blackening seasoning. Allow to sit for at least 15 minutes. Heat medium-sized skillet with coconut oil over medium heat. Once the oil is hot, add the chicken breasts, sprinkle with salt, and cook on each side for 5 minutes or until juices run clear.

Yields 2 servings.

Curried Coconut Chicken

When you cook with curry, it's important to remember to cook it thoroughly or else it can cause stomach upset. It's not just a seasoning you can throw in at the last minute, because it won't taste right or digest properly. This great, simple Thai dish really showcases the flavor of coconut in a savory dish.

- 2 tablespoons virgin coconut oil, divided
- 1 small red onion, thinly sliced
- 4 teaspoons curry powder, divided
- 2 boneless, skinless chicken breasts, cubed into bite-sized pieces
- ¼ cup unsweetened coconut milk
- 1 tablespoon chopped peanuts or scallions for garnish

Heat a large skillet over medium heat. Add 1 tablespoon of the coconut oil and melt. Add the onions and 2 teaspoons of curry powder, and cook for 5 minutes or until the onion starts to become translucent. Using a slotted spoon, remove the onions from the curry juice and set aside.

Add the chicken and the remaining curry powder and coconut oil. Cook for 12 minutes or until the chicken is done and browned. Add the onions to the chicken mix, and then pour in the coconut milk. Simmer for 15 minutes or until the sauce is thickened. Garnish with chopped peanuts or scallions.

Serve over choice of rice.

Yields 2 servings.

Coconut Margherita Pizza

This creamy, luscious dish has it all: the crispy crunch of the crust, the zest of the basil, and the creamy texture of the sauce. You better double the recipe and make two!

- 1 cup unsweetened coconut milk
- 4 cloves garlic, minced
- ½ teaspoon sea salt
- 1 fresh pizza dough (available in the freezer section or in the deli)

- 1 tablespoon virgin coconut oil, melted
- ½ cup fresh basil leaves
- 1 tomato, sliced
- 1/2 teaspoon oregano

Combine coconut milk, garlic, and salt in a saucepan, and cook until it starts to thicken. Press the pizza dough out into a 12- to 14-inch round pan, and brush with the coconut oil. Add the sauce, and then layer the tomatoes and basil over the crust. Sprinkle with oregano, and bake 20 to 25 minutes or until the crust is golden brown.

Yields 4 servings.

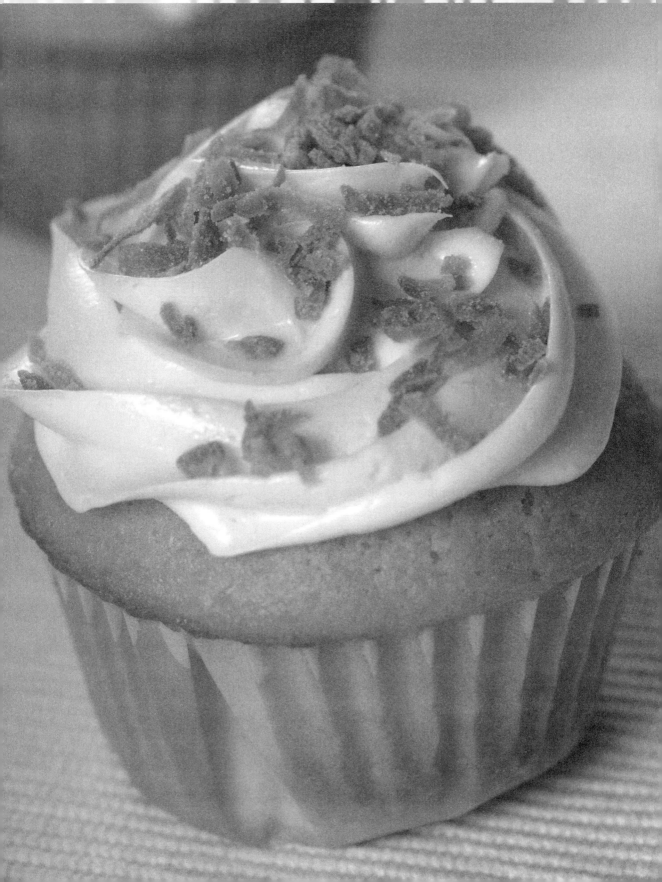

COCONUT OIL RECIPES FOR SNACKS AND DESSERTS

Crispy, Flaky Piecrust

When you replace the standard fats in piecrusts with coconut oil, the results are flaky, tender crusts your grandmother would be proud of. Depending on what you're going to fill it with, you can use either refined or virgin coconut oil. The key to a great crust is to make sure that your water is ice-cold.

- 1½ cups all-purpose flour
- ¼ teaspoon sea salt
- ½ cup coconut oil, either refined or virgin

- 1 egg
- ¼ cup ice water
- 2 teaspoons white vinegar

Combine flour and salt in a medium glass bowl. Add coconut oil and cut it into the flour mixture with a pastry cutter until the mixture is crumbly and even-textured.

Add the egg and knead just until it's mixed in. Quickly add the ice water and vinegar all at once, and knead the dough until it's a cohesive ball.

Divide into half and roll one-half out onto a lightly floured surface until it's ¼ inch thick. Place in pie plate and either add filling or bake. Repeat with the second crust, or freeze it.

Yields 2 piecrusts.

Coconut Oil Buttercream Icing

If most people knew how buttercream icing was made, they would probably never eat it again! All of that butter and lard is a heart attack on a cupcake, but now you don't have to go without frosting. Simply substituting coconut oil for the butter and lard will give you a creamy frosting everyone will love. It's still packed with calories, but at least it's not clogging your arteries!

- 1 cup coconut oil, virgin or refined
- Dash of sea salt
- 3½ cups (approximately) confectioners' sugar

- 2 tablespoons milk or coconut milk
- 1 tablespoon vanilla extract or any extract that you prefer

Put the coconut oil and salt in a bowl, and add the sugar to it slowly, ½ cup at a time. Once all of your sugar is incorporated, add the milk and extract. If the icing is a bit thin, add more sugar. If you'd like to add color, do so at the end so you get a true color.

Yields 3½ cups frosting.

Orange Coconut Cupcakes

These citrusy little delights will be devoured by everybody from kids to retirees. They're great for school parties, or you can add some filling to make elegant cupcakes suitable for a wedding or shower.

- 1 cup virgin coconut oil
- 1 cup granulated sugar
- 3 medium eggs, room temperature
- 2 teaspoons orange zest
- ⅓ teaspoon orange extract
- ¼ cup whole or 2% milk

- 1½ cups all-purpose flour
- ¾ teaspoon baking powder
- ¾ teaspoon baking soda
- ¼ teaspoon sea salt
- ½ cup unsweetened coconut flakes

Preheat oven to 350 degrees F, and line 12 muffin cups with cupcake papers.

In a separate bowl, combine flour, baking powder, baking soda, and salt.

Combine coconut oil, sugar, and eggs in a bowl, and beat until the sugar is dissolved. Add in the orange zest, extract, and milk. Begin adding the dry ingredients (except for the coconut flakes), and continue to mix until well combined. Beat for another minute.

Fill cupcake papers two-thirds full, and bake for 20 minutes or until a toothpick inserted in the middle comes out clean. Cool for 30 minutes and frost with a modified version (use coconut extract) of the Coconut Oil Buttercream Icing presented earlier. Decorate the cupcakes with the coconut flakes.

Yields 12 cupcakes.

Coconut Cream Pie

We couldn't have a coconut oil cookbook without including a recipe for coconut cream pie! Use the Crispy, Flaky Piecrust recipe presented earlier, making it with virgin coconut oil. This pie is creamy and decadent, but you've taken much of the "bad" fat out just by using coconut milk and coconut oil in place of the cream and the butter. You'll never miss them, though!

- 3 cups unsweetened coconut milk
- ½ cup granulated sugar
- 2 egg yolks
- ⅓ cup arrowroot powder
- 1½ teaspoons vanilla extract
- 3 tablespoons virgin coconut oil
- 1¼ cups sweetened shredded coconut, divided

Combine the coconut milk, sugar, egg yolks, arrowroot powder, and vanilla in a heavy-bottomed medium saucepan. Whisk together until smooth and cook over medium heat, stirring constantly until it thickens. Remove from heat, and add the coconut oil and 1 cup of the shredded coconut, stirring until combined. Pour into your homemade coconut crust and sprinkle the remaining coconut over the top of the pie.

Yields 1 pie.

Coconut Lime Bars

These are great snacks for hot afternoons when something refreshing and light is called for. It's also a great dish to take as your dessert to your next potluck. As with all of our desserts, the coconut oil makes these bars much healthier, no matter how you slice them.

- 1¼ cups all-purpose flour
- ¼ cup confectioners' sugar
- ¾ cup virgin coconut oil
- 4 eggs

- 1¼ cups granulated sugar
- ½ cup fresh lime juice
- 1½ teaspoons baking powder
- ½ cup sweetened shredded coconut

Preheat oven to 350 degrees F. Combine the flour, confectioners' sugar, and coconut oil in a small bowl. Mix until it's crumbly in texture, and press into the bottom of a 13 x 9–inch cake pan. This is your crust!

In a medium glass bowl, whisk the eggs and then add the granulated sugar, lime juice, and baking powder. Mix until sugar is dissolved, and then pour into crust. Sprinkle the shredded coconut on top. Bake for 20 to 25 minutes or until it's brown. Remove from oven and allow to cool for at least 30 minutes. Slice into 2-inch squares and enjoy.

Yields about 24 squares.

Crispy Sweet Potato Chips

One of the most difficult processed foods to give up in the quest for better health is often potato chips. These crispy, salty, and slightly sweet chips are a great alternative without the hydrogenated fats, mystery ingredients, and starchy white potatoes.

- 2 sweet potatoes, skinned and sliced as thinly as possible
- 2 tablespoons virgin coconut oil
- 1 teaspoon sea salt
- 1 teaspoon black pepper

Preheat oven to 400 degrees F. In a medium bowl, add the potatoes and drizzle the coconut oil over them. Sprinkle on the salt and pepper and toss to coat. Spread on a cookie sheet greased with coconut oil and bake 25 to 30 minutes or until chips are crispy. If there are leftovers, store in an airtight container.

Yields 4 servings.

Coconut Buckeyes

These traditional little yummies are common in the Appalachians and are typically made with butter. Substituting coconut oil for the butter greatly improves both the texture and the health factor.

- 1 cup creamy peanut butter
- ¼ cup + 1 teaspoon virgin coconut oil, divided
- 2 tablespoons honey
- 1 teaspoon vanilla extract
- 3 cups confectioners' sugar
- 4 ounces semisweet baker's chocolate

Mix the peanut butter, ¼ cup coconut oil, honey, and vanilla in a medium bowl until smooth. Add the confectioners' sugar, ¼ cup at a time, and blend thoroughly before adding more. When it's firm enough to form into balls and hold its shape, stop adding sugar.

Melt the chocolate in the microwave and stir in 1 teaspoon coconut oil.

Line a cookie sheet with aluminum foil. Form the peanut butter mixture into 1½-inch balls and dip into chocolate. Set on the cookie sheet and allow to set.

Yields about 25 buckeyes.

Strawberry Coconut Muffins

These are good for a snack or even for breakfast on the run. If you'd like to really make them healthy, try using coconut flour in place of regular flour. The coconut oil adds not only a nice flavor, but also a beautiful golden color and a crisp crown.

- 3 cups all-purpose flour
- 1 teaspoon baking powder
- ½ teaspoon baking soda
- ½ teaspoon salt
- ½ cup virgin coconut oil
- 1¼ cup granulated sugar

- 4 medium eggs
- 1 teaspoon vanilla extract
- 1 cup unsweetened coconut milk
- 1 cup fresh strawberries, capped and sliced
- ½ cup sweetened shredded coconut

Preheat oven to 350 degrees F, and line 12 muffin cups with cupcake papers.

Combine flour, baking powder, baking soda, and salt in a smaller bowl and set aside.

In a large glass mixing bowl, cream together coconut oil and sugar until sugar is dissolved. Add eggs in one at a time, and then mix in the vanilla. Add the flour mixture and mix until combined. Slowly start adding the coconut milk until it's all in the batter. Gently fold in the strawberries. Add the batter to muffin cups, filling each one about two-thirds of the way full. Sprinkle with shredded coconut.

Bake for 18 to 22 minutes or until crowns are golden. Remove from oven and cool.

Yields 12 muffins.

Modified Coconut Hummus Dip

Though the traditional recipe for hummus is healthy and delicious, we felt like a coconut oil substitute might be good just for fun!

- 1 can chickpeas, drained
- 1 tablespoon virgin coconut oil
- 2 cloves garlic, minced
- 1 tablespoon sun-dried tomatoes
- ½ teaspoon salt

Put the chickpeas in your food processor and blend for at least 1 minute or until smooth and fluffy. Add each of the next four ingredients one at a time, and mix for 1 minute in between each addition. This may sound like a lot of mixing, but it's necessary! When everything is combined, store in an airtight container in the fridge.

Yields about 1 cup.

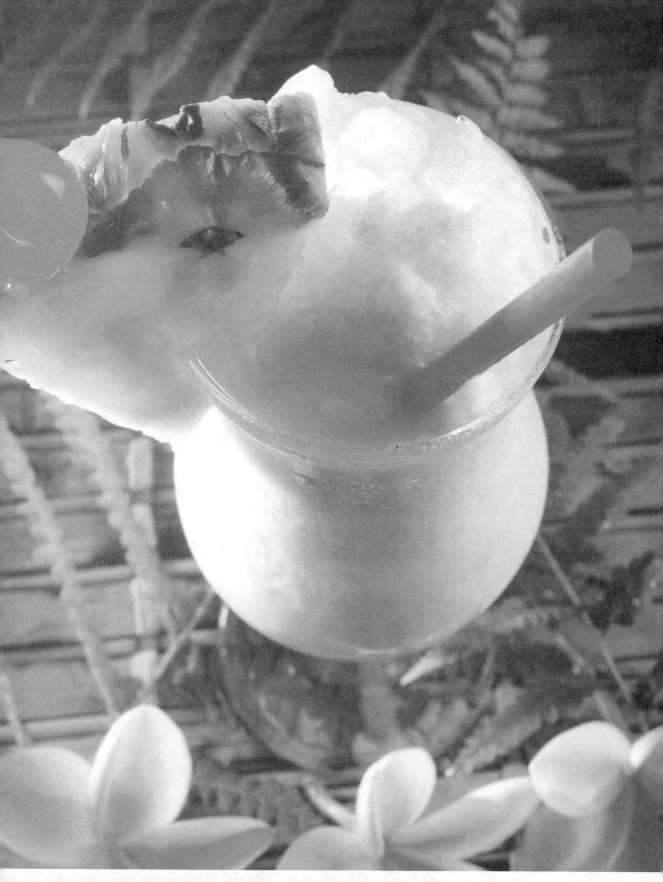

COCONUT OIL RECIPES FOR BEVERAGES

Creamy, Dreamy Cocoa

Fresh, homemade hot cocoa brings back memories of cold nights, sledding adventures, and holiday mornings spent with family, but hardly anybody makes hot cocoa from scratch anymore. This creamy, comforting rendition will make your heart as happy as your taste buds.

- 2 cups milk, 2 percent or light coconut
- 1 tablespoon virgin coconut oil
- 2 tablespoons cocoa powder
- 2 tablespoons granulated sugar or honey, or to taste
- 1 teaspoon vanilla extract

Place the milk and the coconut oil in a medium saucepan over medium heat. Whisk in the cocoa powder and the sugar, and bring to a simmer. Simmer for 1 minute or until sugar is dissolved. Stir in vanilla and serve in mugs.

Yields 2 servings.

Coconut-Hazelnut Coffee Creamer

Flavored coffee creamers are one of life's little guilty pleasures that many people sacrifice in the name of health and wellness. The commercial ones are packed full of chemicals and hydrogenated fats that just don't make the taste worth it, but now you don't have to settle for them.

- 1 can sweetened coconut milk (14 ounces), room temperature
- ½ tablespoon vanilla extract
- 1 teaspoon hazelnut extract
- 1 tablespoon virgin coconut oil, melted

You'll need to use a whisk or the blender for this because you want to make an emulsion. It may also help if the coconut milk is a bit warmer than room temperature. Put the coconut milk and the extracts in your blender, and turn it on the low setting. Slowly begin to drizzle in the coconut oil until it's completely added, and then blend for another 30 seconds. Store in a bottle in the fridge for up to a week, but it's doubtful it will last that long!

Yields about 2 cups.

Coconut Spiced Tea

Spicy and just a bit exotic, this tea is great for a cold afternoon or as an afternoon pick-me-up. The caffeine in the tea and the MCTs in the coconut oil will have you back at full steam in no time at all. Plus it tastes great.

- 1 cup water
- 1 cup unsweetened coconut milk
- 2 standard tea bags or 2 teaspoons loose black tea
- 1 teaspoon virgin coconut oil
- ⅛ teaspoon ground ginger
- ⅛ teaspoon ground nutmeg
- ⅛ teaspoon ground allspice
- ⅛ teaspoon ground cinnamon

Bring water and coconut milk to a simmer in a medium saucepan. Remove from heat and add tea. Allow to steep for 3 to 5 minutes and then remove tea bags. Stir in the coconut oil and the rest of the spices. The coconut milk has a natural sweetness, but if you'd like it sweeter, use your sweetener of choice.

Yields 2 cups.

Moroccan Spiced Latte

This robust chai-like coffee experience tastes great and wakes you right up. The flavors combine to take you on a vacation to lands faraway, and the coconut flavor lends just the right amount of nuttiness.

- 2 espresso shots
- 8 ounces unsweetened coconut milk
- 1 teaspoon virgin coconut oil
- ½ teaspoon cinnamon
- 1 dash ground cloves
- 1 dash ground cardamom
- 1 dash ground nutmeg
- 1 dash ground ginger
- 1 dash ground black pepper

Make your espresso as you usually would and pour into a cappuccino cup. Steam the coconut milk and coconut oil together, then whisk in the spices. Pour over the espresso and enjoy.

Yields 1 serving.

Virgin Piña Colada

We couldn't write a book on coconut oil without including a piña colada recipe any more than we could have left out the coconut cream pie. This one has a bit of an unexpected twist, so be ready!

- ½ cup sweetened coconut milk
- ½ cup unsweetened coconut milk
- 1 cup pineapple juice
- 2 teaspoons molasses, preferably blackstrap
- 1½ cups ice
- 1 tablespoon virgin coconut oil, melted
- 2 pineapple wedges

Put the coconut milks, pineapple juice, molasses, and ice in the blender, and blend on low for 15 seconds. Then switch up to medium. Slowly drizzle the coconut oil into the slush to avoid clumps. Pour into two hurricane glasses and garnish with the pineapple.

Yields 2 servings.

Goombay Smash Smoothie

We've taken one of the best beach cocktails ever and turned it into a power smoothie! When you taste it, you'll want to trade your morning run for a rousing game of beach volleyball! The fiber, complex carbohydrates, and MCTs make it the perfect pre- or post-workout drink, too.

- ½ cup unsweetened coconut milk
- 1 apricot
- ½ cup pineapple chunks
- ½ banana
- 1 teaspoon molasses
- ¼ cup orange juice
- 5 ice cubes
- 1 tablespoon virgin coconut oil, melted

Place all ingredients except the coconut oil in your blender and blend on low. As it mixes, turn to medium and begin to slowly drizzle in the coconut oil. Blend until smooth and enjoy.

Yields about 2 cups.

Chocolate Coconut Weight-Loss Smoothie

Cocoa is a proven metabolism stimulator, so when you combine it with the furnace-revving power of coconut oil and the staying power of protein, you've got a healthy, delicious drink that helps you lose weight and beat the sweet cravings at the same time.

- 1 cup unsweetened coconut milk
- 1 tablespoon almond butter
- 2 teaspoons cocoa powder
- 1 tablespoon honey or maple syrup
- 4 ice cubes
- 1 tablespoon virgin coconut oil

Place all ingredients except the coconut oil in the blender and blend until smooth. Slowly drizzle in the coconut oil until combined. Enjoy.

Yields 1 serving.

Green Island Delight

Getting used to drinking anything green can be a bit of an adjustment, but after one sip of this one, you're going to be hooked. It's rich in antioxidants, healthy enzymes, phytonutrients, and all the good stuff coconut oil brings to the table. Drink up!

- 2 cups fresh spinach
- ½ cup fresh pineapple, cubed
- 1 banana
- 2 kiwis, peeled

- 1 cup unsweetened coconut milk
- 4 or 5 ice cubes
- 1 tablespoon virgin coconut oil, melted

Add everything but the coconut oil to your blender and start on low. Once it starts to mix well, switch to medium and begin to slowly drizzle in the coconut oil. Once everything is added, enjoy "going green"!

Yields 1 serving.

Cocoberry Smoothie

Some drinks are just for fun, and this is one of them . . . or at least that's what the kids will think. The berries provide a nice antioxidant punch, and the banana is packed with potassium and calcium. We need say no more when it comes to the coconut oil.

- 1 cup raspberries
- 1 cup strawberries
- 1 cup unsweetened coconut milk
- 4 or 5 ice cubes
- 1 tablespoon virgin coconut oil, melted

Add all ingredients except the coconut oil to your blender, and mix on low speed until it starts to get smooth. Switch to medium and slowly drizzle in the coconut oil. Pour into a glass and enjoy!

Yields about 2 cups.

Coconut Mornings

One of the best things that you can do for your body is to give it a nutritious start to the day. Without proper fuel, your brain can't function and your muscles won't perform optimally, either. You wouldn't run your car on empty, so don't run your body with no fuel! This smoothie will get your motor running and your gears turning without a ton of empty calories or harmful chemicals.

- ¼ cup rolled oats
- 1 tablespoon almond butter
- 2 teaspoons molasses
- 1 scoop egg white protein powder
- 2 teaspoons cocoa powder
- 1 banana
- ½ cup unsweetened coconut milk
- 2 or 3 ice cubes
- 1 tablespoon virgin coconut oil, melted

Add all ingredients except the coconut oil to your blender. Blend on low until the mixture starts to blend well. At this point if it's a bit thick, add an extra ¼ cup of coconut milk or water. Once it has a good consistency, switch to medium speed and begin to add the coconut oil in a drizzle. Blend until mixed and enjoy.

Yields 1 serving.

CONCLUSION

Throughout the pages of this book, we've touched on some of the most useful benefits of coconut oil, but we didn't cover everything. As with many holistic and natural treatments, coconut oil was used for millennia before people understood how it worked. To our ancestors, it didn't matter what the chemistry was behind it; all that mattered was that it was effective for what they needed it for.

Once we started taking things apart to see how they work, we entered the age of "smart" medicine, and those who supposedly had it all figured out declared that saturated fats were killers. Ages of practical evidence were washed away by a couple of half-formed experiments that didn't even use virgin coconut oil to arrive at their erroneous conclusions.

Twenty years later, researchers are just now beginning to admit that perhaps they shouldn't have made such a blanket statement regarding saturated fats. Medium-chain triglycerides have received a clean bill of health, and coconut oil is back on the table and in the pantry where it belongs.

We hope that you've enjoyed learning about some of the basic uses of coconut oil and that you get much use out of the recipes that we've shared. Until next time, good health and happy eating!

GLOSSARY

Antimicrobial—A broad term referring to an agent that kills some type of microorganism. Typically, agents are assigned a category based on the type of microorganism that they kill, i.e., antibiotics, antifungals, and antivirals.

Antioxidant—An agent that prevents oxidation by binding with the free radical and thus stabilizing it without causing harm to any other cells. Oxidation in the body causes everything from wrinkles to dry skin and even cancer.

Arrowroot powder—A white powder made from the starchy root of several different tropical plants. It's often used as a healthier alternative to cornstarch and is an excellent thickening agent.

Castile soap—A natural, olive-oil-based soap that's often used as the base for homemade soaps, shampoos, and other cleansing agents. Because it's often concentrated, you shouldn't use it without diluting it.

Cholesterol—A type of fat made in the liver from dietary fat and used by the body to build and maintain cell membranes and moderate permeability of cells. You need it in moderate amounts, but in excess, it contributes to atherosclerosis and heart disease.

Coconut cream—The thick, nonliquid substance that separates and rises to the top while coconut milk and coconut oil are being made. Cream of coconut is coconut cream that's been sweetened.

Coconut flour—Flour made from finely grinding dried coconut meat. It is great for baking.

Coconut milk—Made by boiling coconut meat and water, then allowing a "setting" period while the milk and cream separate. Often used by vegans, health enthusiasts, cooks, and coconut enthusiasts as a milk replacement.

Coconut water—The thin liquid found in the center of a coconut when you crack it open. It's a rich source of nutrients.

Essential oils—Typically extracted by a distillation process from the parent plant, essential oils contain the distinctive smell and healing characteristics, or essence, of that plant. Though sometimes edible, essential oils can also be poisonous. They're used for a wide variety of homeopathic purposes, including massage, aromatherapy, etc. Also called *volatile oils* or *ethereal oils*.

Extracts—Obtained by simply pressing, macerating, or soaking the "juices" out of a plant for sensory use, including flavorings and scents. They don't necessarily contain the medicinal or chemical qualities of a plant like essential oils do.

Free radical—An atom that has lost an electron due to a weak bond and is now unstable. It doesn't "like" to exist in an unstable state and will steal electrons from other atoms in an attempt to become stable again. This starts a chain reaction that eventually damages or even kills cells and causes such issues as aging, poor skin, disease, and cancer.

HDL cholesterol—Short for *high-density lipoprotein*, HDL is the good type of cholesterol that cruises the bloodstream and picks up excess bad cholesterol and escorts it out of the body.

LDL cholesterol—Short for *low-density lipoprotein*, LDL is the bad type of cholesterol that deposits on the insides of your arteries and is later oxidized and made toxic by white blood cells. This leads to atherosclerosis and cardiovascular disease.

Lipids—Naturally occurring waxes, sterols, fat-soluble vitamins, fats including triglycerides, fatty acids, and other molecules that perform such functions as energy storage and cell signaling, and make up the outer protective cell membranes.

Metabolism—The process by which your body performs chemical processes to sustain life. Most people simplify this process to relate it to weight loss and think of it as how fast your body burns calories. That's actually only a small part of the entire metabolic process, and the correct term for that part of the metabolic process is called *catabolism*.

Smoke point—The temperature at which a fat starts to burn and smoke. Once it smokes, the flavor is typically ruined.

Trans fats—A type of unsaturated fat that has trans-isomer fatty acids. They're found in extremely small amounts in some meats, but the vast majority of them are created during the process that turns liquid vegetable oils into solids. They turn to sludge in your arteries and raise bad cholesterols without raising the good ones. They're so bad that the FDA requires trans fats to be listed on labels.